What Really Happens After Childbirth

....

A candid tell-all about the physical and emotional changes I experienced after having my babies.

Robin Anderson

Foreword by Dr. Brad Chesney, OB/GYN

Cover Illustration by ***Norris Hall***

Cover Design by ***Wax Family Printing***

ISBN: 978-0-9815604-2-7

Mom Life Publishing

PO Box 10284

Murfreesboro, TN 37129

Acknowledgements

Thank you to everyone who encouraged me to move forward with this project. I was so passionate about sharing this information while I was recording these thoughts. Many times since, I have struggled with whether or not this was something to be shared outside the circle of my personal friends and family. Thank you to all my friends who believed my story would help others through this crazy wonderful time in their own lives. So glad you didn't think I was absolutely nuts for wanting to air all my personal issues! Thank you to my sister in law, Dana, for transferring my voice recordings so I was able to use them to finish this book. Thank you Kendrah for your final review and the encouragement to get this book published "one way or another."

Thank you to Dr. Kimberly McGowan and Dr. Brad Chesney for delivering my beautiful babies safely into this world. Thank you to the labor and delivery staff at St. Thomas Rutherford Hospital for making my hospital experience so positive. A special thank you to those amazing physicians and nurses in the NICU caring for our sweet baby boy. Thank you to Women's Health Specialists and the Murfreesboro Medical Clinic for your compassion and support during my pregnancies. Thank you to Dr. Brad Chesney for taking the time to review my manuscript and the kind words of inspiration. Thank you for believing that my story could help patients getting ready to embark on this journey for the first time.

I appreciate and thank Susan Gall, copy editor, for taking the time to review a manuscript from a mom on a mission to self-publish. Thank you for your suggestions and corrections to my manuscript that so desperately needed help with grammar and punctuation. Thank you to Norris Hall for providing the cover illustration. I am grateful to have an original Norris Hall illustration and am amazed at your artistic talent. I am so pleased with your interpretation of a mom facing all the crazy issues after childbirth.

Thank you to Weston Wax and the wonderful team at Wax Family Printing for the time and patience spent working with me to develop the cover and interior design. I am so thankful to Jeremy Isbell for seeing my vision and understanding my enthusiasm. Thank you to Sarah Monroe, graphic designer, for her creativity and expertise. I stopped in Wax Family Printing one day for something completely unrelated and walked out knowing I had found a way to develop my manuscript into a book. Thank you for making my book a reality.

Thank you to my sister, Michelle, for listening and guiding me when I need it the most. And, thank you for being the best sister and friend I could imagine! Thank you to my parents, Harley and Linda Foutch, for teaching me to always finish what you start and to chase my dreams. Thank you for the life lessons you have taught me and continue to teach me every day. Thank you to my in-laws, Roger and Rhoda Anderson, for loving me as their own daughter. Ryan and I are blessed to have parents who have shown us amazing examples of marriage and devotion.

Most of all, thank you to Ryan. I have spent many late nights working on this project. You have been nothing but supportive in the years it has taken to develop this book. You never thought I was crazy for wanting to share my most intimate issues about childbirth. I appreciate that you had no reservations about me including your own struggles during the hardest time of our lives. You are an unbelievable husband and I am so proud to be married to you. Thank you for always making me laugh! I love you and I can't wait to spend the rest of my life with you!

Thank you to my three silly, creative, and wonderful kiddos. I love you Ashlyn, Katie Ryan, and Brady. You have given me the most precious times of my life. I am so grateful God blessed our family with each of you. Thank you for being my inspiration and the greatest gifts your dad and I could ever imagine. I love being your mommy!

Contents

Foreword

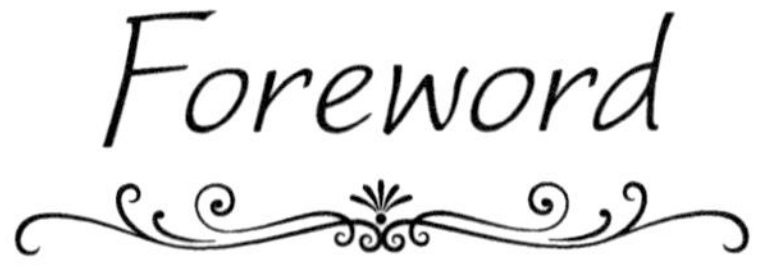

It's not every day that one of my patients comes in for an appointment and tells me that they have written a book about the trials and tribulations of the postpartum period. When Robin explained the subject matter, I told her to bring me a copy of the manuscript! Robin has captured a very unique time in a mother's life. Her story gives details that are usually not discussed or even considered during pregnancy. As an OB/GYN, I am focused on the health of the mother and her baby throughout the pregnancy and delivery. Throughout the pregnancy, our practice is here for support and to answer any questions along the way.

There are always unique situations, but on average an OB patient has thirteen doctor's visits during her pregnancy. As long as there are no major complications, there is usually one six-week follow-up appointment that occurs post-hospital discharge. We have had thirteen times throughout the pregnancy to answer questions and for the mother to voice her concerns. It is logistically impossible to provide the same support for a mom in the days and weeks after delivery. The hospital I am affiliated with does a very good job at offering a class to moms, before they are discharged, about what physical changes to expect after giving birth. This class covers several of the topics that are mentioned in this book. However, the 30- to 45-minute class is so brief and overwhelming that it is hard to retain the information that is given.

Robin offers a candid view of some of the things that you may go through during the postpartum period and beyond. I am excited that this book gives women an opportunity to understand what may happen after their own labor and delivery. I am glad that Robin is willing to share these intimate issues and struggles with other women. In so doing, she has truly captured the essence of the postpartum period. I sincerely hope that all of my patients who are first-time mothers have the opportunity to read this before baby arrives!

Dr. Brad Chesney

Introduction

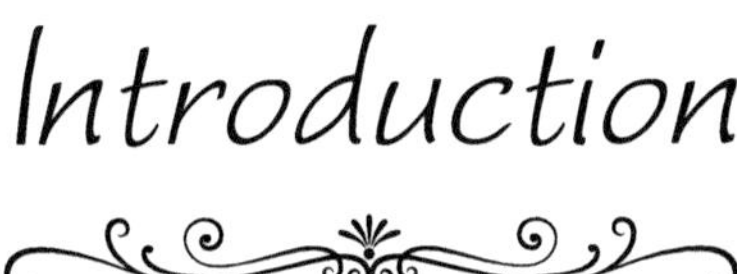

This is not a pregnancy book. It's not a book about getting your body back in shape after having a baby. It's not a parenting book or a book about bringing your baby home. This is not typical of what you will read about in most books concerning pregnancy and childbirth. This book is about what happens to your body immediately following childbirth. It is about the very short period of time right after you give birth that nobody talks about before you have your baby. I'm not clinical, so this book isn't in medical terms. It's just a book filled with the details you talk about with your girlfriends right after you have a baby and wish that you would have known beforehand. I intentionally didn't research the proper terminology or collaborate with a nurse or doctor because I wanted you to hear it from one girlfriend to another.

This is the insanely personal account of what I experienced soon after I gave birth to my third child. I use the term *insanely personal* because after looking back at the details I gave at the time, it kind of freaks me out that I am sharing all this with the world. I am writing this book from voice recordings I made while I was going through that time in my life. I'm not sure what gave me the idea to do this, but I am so glad I did. It has been almost two years now since my youngest child was born. There is no way I could write about dealing with your body after childbirth now in the same way as I did when I was actually going through it. I know I couldn't explain everything with the same clarity and detail as I did then. And at the time, my inhibitions were gone, so what I wrote was exactly how I felt. When you have just had a baby you will tell anyone anything about it in full detail, or at least I would! Now, two years after the fact, I'm a little more discreet about it all, and I can't remember it well enough to even give the same perspective.

This book came about in the middle of the night when I was nursing my baby boy. At the time, I had just had a C-section and was going through all the lovely things that come with the recovery. While I was up feeding my baby, I had a thought. I knew I would never again be able to readily account for what I was experiencing at that moment, so I grabbed a pen and paper. The beginning of this book was actually written on a scrap of paper. I started to get my feelings down as soon as I got my son back to sleep. I worked on it until I couldn't keep my eyes open anymore, and then I continued again the next night. I was frustrated with having only these small bits of time to get these thoughts down on paper. Then I had the idea of using a voice recorder; this opened up the opportunity to get my feelings recorded at whatever moment I could find the time to speak into the recorder.

I was trying my best to get everything documented while I was still on maternity leave and before I lost it all in the "baby fog." We will talk more about that in the book. Anyway, remember, this was my third child. I had a five year old and a two year old at the time also. Not much free time going on in my world. I was recording all this on the voice recorder on my cell phone, which was always with me. These recordings would happen whenever and wherever I had the chance. Some moms in the elementary school car line would look at me a little funny in the car. I don't know why because so many people use hands-free devices in the car. I couldn't have looked that out of the ordinary. Maybe it's because I talk with my hands so much. Anyone who knows me personally knows how much I talk with my hands. When I am really excited about a topic, it's just exaggerated that much more. I couldn't be any more passionate about getting this info to "moms to be" out there, so I bet my hands were going wild.

I have many recordings from middle-of-the-night breastfeeding moments. It's so much easier to use a voice recorder instead of writing when you are trying to nurse or give your baby a bottle! I would record while I was in the shower, in the car, doing dishes, and everything else you could imagine a mom of three kids five and younger might be doing. My favorites are the recordings that have the kids yelling in the background. I was probably hiding out to try and finish my thought process before I got back to my kiddos. If this is your first pregnancy, you will soon understand. We moms have "hiding places" where we can at least get an important phone call in without being interrupted.

This is how I captured the moments when a new mom is going through all the "stuff" everybody leaves out in the pregnancy books. I thought I had it rougher than any new mom in the world because nobody told me about all this! As I will explain soon, it's not that everyone means to keep you in the dark; they just don't fully remember! Even your mom, best friend, sister, and all the people who are the very closest to you can't fully explain it to you. Today, when my youngest isn't even two yet, I can no longer explain it in the same way. This is my gift to you. This is me sharing with you all my memories of that time. The best part about it is, they aren't *memories*. They are just what happened while it was happening. Not sure why God gave me the insight to do this because it's God who designed every new mom to forget about it all so quick. I'm thinking it's because He knows how weirded out I got about everything and is giving me a chance to save others from experiencing the same feeling.

I don't know how most authors write books, and this is my first and probably only one. But I am actually writing this introduction before I write the book. Well, I guess that's not all true, because my book is already written—it's just not on paper yet. What I mean is, I am intentionally writing the introduction before I start in on the voice recordings. I want to keep these recordings just as I made them initially. Yes, I will actually turn them into full sentences and tweak them here and there so they make more sense, but I want to hold myself accountable to keeping them as they were recorded. I'm thinking if I tell you up front that I promise to account for each detail just as vividly as I recorded, then I actually will. This is exciting and terrifying all at once. I haven't shared many of these details with my husband and never intended to. I feel very strongly that your spouse does not and should not know everything about having babies. He should be very supportive but save the nitty gritty for your girlfriends!

You may be wondering why it has taken me so long to actually write this book when I have been so excited about the idea. If you have three kids, you aren't wondering! It is so hard to keep up with work and family that a book had to remain on the back burner. Now I am determined to make this book happen. Today is July 8, and I have given myself until the end of the summer to finish this. My husband, Ryan, works second shift, so my plan is to write every evening when the kids go to bed until he gets home. I let my kids stay up late, but we may have to work on earlier bedtimes the rest of the summer. I should have at least two hours every night. I am so ready to get this book written! Thank you for giving me the chance to share with you some of the absolute best and hardest days of my life.

I am concentrating on what happened to me after delivery, but nobody can resist telling their labor and delivery story. Moms rank this as their best accomplishment ever, as we should! We birthed a baby; something you dream about and are completely terrified of your entire life. While you are pregnant, you hear everyone's victory story. I love to hear moms tell about the birth of their children. Whether scheduled or spur of the moment, vaginal, or C-section, natural or not, we all have a story! We all experience different levels of it being uncomfortable, painful, terrifying, exciting, joyous, emotional, and surreal all at once! No matter how easy or hard it actually was, *your baby* was born! It's the greatest miracle that will ever happen to you, and in the midst of your story, you will experience the happiest tears you have ever cried!

Here are my stories. . .

First Baby—We went to the hospital the night before I was supposed to be induced. This was a couple days after my actual due date. They gave me Cytotec, a medication that was supposed to help start contractions, and hooked me up to an IV. The contractions never got strong, so first thing in the morning they came in and broke my water. It didn't take long with Pitocin, the most common drug to induce labor, to get my contractions going. They quickly got very strong. I remember asking for my epidural, and was told it was too early but they gave me something to cut the pain of the contractions. I continued to have strong contractions for a while. They finally got my epidural in and kicked up the Pitocin. I didn't respond well to the Pitocin, so they had to turn it down and put me on oxygen. It took all day for me to fully dilate. They kept me on oxygen until I had finally dilated to a ten and it was time to push. I always heard just a couple pushes and the baby is out. *Wrong!* I pushed for what seemed like forever, but I don't think it was much more than an hour. When it was time to push, my epidural was no longer working, and it was too late to get more. I had complete control over my movements and felt extreme pain and pressure. Finally, with nurses on top of me pushing my knees to my chest and me pushing like crazy, my sweet little girl was born at 7:17 pm. She was 8 pounds and 5 ounces, and as soon as I held that sweet baby with completely unexpected jet black hair, I was smitten! It didn't matter how long and hard the day had been. Mission accomplished. We became parents and nothing else mattered!

Second Baby—My original due date was on December 25, 2009. Oops! Ryan and I sure didn't mean to do that. We were trying for months, but didn't do the math to determine when the baby would be due. I was determined to not have that baby on Christmas Day! Who can compete with Jesus' Birthday? December birthdays are hard enough! I was huge and so ready to deliver. We were trying to figure out what would work best with my doctor's schedule. They offered induction and I jumped on it. I had said I wasn't going to induce because I did not respond well to Pitocin and I wanted to experience my body going into labor naturally, but once again I was on a schedule. We decided on December 22. The night before induction I was wrapping Christmas presents in our living room and started having major contractions. I thought I might be going into labor anyway, but they subsided quickly. This time we went to the hospital first thing in the morning, thank goodness! They immediately broke my water and got me started on Pitocin. Second baby, so I thought I'd have that baby by noon. Not the case. I dilated a little bit quicker this time and thankfully didn't have to be on oxygen, but nobody knew what was coming! My epidural was working very well, thank God! I could feel pressure but that was pretty much it. In the delivery room, they said they could tell she was a big baby, but everyone was surprised at just how big she actually was. Our precious 11-pound baby girl was born at 4:55 pm.

Third Baby—I was monitored very closely during my pregnancy with this baby. At the twenty-week ultrasound when we got the surprising news we were having a boy, we also got the news that he had kidney troubles. It's called hydronephrosis (kidney blockage), meaning one of his kidneys was significantly larger than the other. This is fairly common, especially in boys, and usually they outgrow it while still in utero. It usually happens just because everything isn't growing at the same pace. Our sweet little man's kidney troubles just got worse with every ultrasound. The high-risk obstetrician did not know whether or not he would need surgery shortly after birth, but decided to bring him two weeks early because it was only getting worse and she did not want me to worry about having another gigantic baby. My regular obstetrician agreed, and once again I had an induction date set on the calendar. I went in at thirty-eight weeks, supposedly full term, but our baby wasn't ready to be born yet. We went into the hospital at the crack of dawn, and soon after they broke my water and started the Pitocin. I was given an epidural; given it was my third baby, you would think that I would have dilated quickly, but it didn't happen this time, either. They kept checking me and I showed very little progress. Soon our baby boy's heart rate dropped significantly and the decision was made for an emergency C-section. I didn't care how he got here; I just wanted my baby here safe. They prepped me and gave me the additional pain meds, and then off to surgery. It seemed like it took awhile in the operating room to finally get him delivered, but I know it wasn't long at all. I was just so worried that he was in distress, and we weren't getting him out quick enough. Our 7-pound, 5-ounce adorable baby boy was born at 8:04 pm.

If you are pregnant or just recently had your baby, congratulations! Thank you for taking this precious time in your life to read *one mom's experience* with hopes to make it a little easier for you. I am so privileged to be a part of these amazing moments. If you are a new dad or dad-to-be, please stop reading now. This is way too embarrassing for me to think that some random guy I don't know is about to know way too much about all of my issues! Or, if you aren't a random guy and I do know you, I *really* need you to stop reading! Trust me guys, you don't want to know all the details. So here goes at telling you just what happened to my body after the miracle of childbirth. I will do my best to transfer the thoughts from my recordings directly on paper without my censorship getting in the way.

Chapter 1

The Idea

Right now it is 12:00 am and I am up with my three-week-old baby boy. He's my third child, my first baby boy. I just finished feeding him; now I am listening to him make sweet baby sounds wondering how long it is going to take him to get back to sleep. I just decided to write this book. I am in a daybed sleeping beside him in the nursery these days and enjoying every moment, even when I get no sleep and am up all night. I did not enjoy this time with my first child and I wished those first few months away. I am soaking up every second of this stage now because I know just how quick it goes. While on maternity leave, I had big hopes of cleaning out closets, organizing all my kids "stuff," and doing home improvements. All of my projects will have to wait. I'm going to focus on writing this book instead.

This book is about your body after having a baby. Most pregnancy books walk you through the entire pregnancy month by month, even week by week. When I was pregnant with my first child, I read lots of them! They tell you just what to expect with what is happening with your body and your baby's development. You can know every detail of what is happening with the miracle growing inside you. We track the changes happening with our own body and know just what symptoms we will have even before they surface. We know how our boobs will change and feel. We learn about stretch marks, cravings, contractions, and hormones. Most moms-to-be learn as much about pregnancy as possible so they understand what is happening to their body while they are going through this amazing journey of motherhood.

Most pregnancy books give you all this detail up until forty weeks. Most talk about actual childbirth and give delivery options and details, but this is the last chapter. You get to forty weeks, deliver your baby, and there's no more insight as to what is to come. Nothing fully prepares you for what to expect with your body *after* childbirth. It's my goal to change that! This was the hardest part for me, and everyone forgets to focus on it! Yes, there may be a checklist for what to take to the hospital and brief descriptions of labor and delivery, but no more precise details. Those days and weeks right after delivery never get the attention they need. This is when we need the details the most!

When you stop and think about it, this is when your body is going through the most change of the entire process. It's taken nine months (really ten months) for your body to go through the pregnancy and changes that take place to give this little baby a safe, comfortable home to grow. Your body grows and adjusts gradually to prepare. There has been a human being living inside you all this time. Now, on one amazing day, that baby is introduced to the world. Your body freaks out afterward! It has not been able to prepare for no longer caring for this little human. There's no step-down process. You are shocked, frustrated, sore, and emotional all at the same time. One day the baby is in your womb and the next you are holding him or her in your arms. Your body and mind need time to recover and get back to a new state of normal. We've got this newborn baby who we love, but he or she is still somewhat of a stranger in our home. We are adjusting, our husbands are adjusting, and our body is left a bizarre mess!

And did I mention our emotions have just had whiplash? All the hormone levels in our body are riding the waves of new motherhood. You are happy and sad and tired all at the same time. I've always thought of myself as an emotionally stable human being. That does not exist with a new mom. I don't care how much you think you have it together; at some point you will be reminded that your emotions are haywire. I remember my sister telling me that right after she had her first baby that she was crying because she missed the feeling of him in her belly. My very supportive brother-in-law couldn't make sense of it. He was trying to explain that the baby was right here for her to love on and hold. He couldn't understand what was wrong with her. She was blubbering about not feeling little kicks anymore and their baby was five feet away from her, happy and healthy. I can so relate now. Who knows what is going to set you off emotionally. At least our hubbies are still in the "I don't know how to say anything right, so I just won't say much stage" from dealing with us during pregnancy, so they aren't shocked when you are ticked or crying or laughing for no apparent reason.

Ask any mom who has had a child longer than two years ago about the first few weeks and you won't get much detail. They will say "It's not that bad," or they will talk about adjusting to having a new baby in the home. It's God's haze keeping them from remembering all the craziness. Ask a brand new mom what is happening with her boobs or how her first pee was after a vaginal delivery, and you will get details! I want to give everyone all the information I can about what you and your body will go through. I have to tell all you first-time mommas that you are not alone. What you experience the first couple of weeks after becoming a mom is normal. We all go through it to some degree, and you need to know what will happen before you are right in the thick of it. This time period is very short in the big scheme of things, and much shorter than pregnancy, but when you are going through it, it seems like *forever*! I'm determined to get the word out before my recall becomes foggy and I forget all the crazy details.

It's not that your friends or family are trying to hide something from you. I think moms actually forget just what they went through. Those memories get mixed in with the whole childbirth memory, which becomes very hazy shortly after you live through it. This is not an accident; this is God's way of making sure siblings exist. This is how God ensures we will continue to procreate even after we've gone through the trauma of childbirth.

This book is not intended to scare you or try to keep you from having kids, although certain parts may come in handy during your daughter's teenage years to deter pregnancy. I've heard of parents using childbirth videos as a way to teach their daughters to practice abstinence. This book just might have the same effect! Every discomfort and every pain is so worth holding the little miracle God has brought into your life. And I, like so many other moms, put myself through it time and time again to experience the extreme joy of motherhood. What is in store for your body is not fun, but it's over quickly, and you *will* get your body and your sexuality back. Maybe not the exact body you had before kids, but it will feel like yours once again.

My first two kids were born by vaginal delivery and my third by C-section. After having two vaginal births, I never dreamed my third would end up in C-section, but that experience has now prepared me to tell you the difference and what to expect after experiencing both. God has blessed my husband and I with three amazing children, but getting them here was not easy. My sister and mom had very quick and easy deliveries. You would think I would, too, but that wasn't the case. My pregnancies were always easy, but labor and deliveries were long and very difficult.

My three kids weighed 8 pounds and 5 ounces, 11 pounds even, and 7 pounds and 5 ounces. Yeah, that's right, I said 11 pounds. Everyone thought it was a misprint when we first got the details out. I'm 5 feet 1 inch tall and usually about 130 pounds, so everyone, including me, was surprised. And no, the 11-pounder was not the C-section. I gave the weights in proper birth order. The smallest of all three ended up being the C-section. That's right, I gave birth to an 11-pound baby vaginally! After she was born and everyone asked how much she weighed, people couldn't help but ask what type of delivery she was. Thank God this was my second child! I actually recovered quicker and easier than after my first.

So, after having three kids including two girls and a boy and experiencing both vaginal and C-section deliveries ranging from 7 to 11 pound babies, why can't I be an expert on the subject? I forgot to mention that my youngest was in the NICU (neonatal intensive-care unit). He was induced two weeks early, and his lungs weren't quite ready so he spent some time in the NICU with oxygen and a feeding tube. So, if needed, I've got you covered there, too. I hope that you do not have to experience this; it's one of the hardest things I've ever been through! We'll talk about that lots more later, just in case you find yourself in this position.

I'm not sure why the time immediately following childbirth is so overlooked. All moms go through it, but we are just left to figure it out as it comes. You take this sweet baby home, but lose yourself in the process for a very short period of time. I want to prepare you the best I can with hopes that you will not be so overwhelmed with what is happening to your body that you are not able to enjoy this precious baby you just welcomed into the world.

Before it's too late, this is something you have to know. Do not clue your hubby in on everything! Now, don't get me wrong. I'm only talking about what happens after you give birth. Your man needs to be a part of the entire pregnancy and delivery. My husband, Ryan, was right beside me every step of the way. You can both see obvious changes happening with your body. Your belly is stretching and your boobs are huge (very exciting if that's not your norm, like me!). Make sure your hubby enjoys your big boobs while he can because they are probably very short lived. The only problem is that as you get further along in your pregnancy, lots of men get weirded out by the whole "our child is in there" thing and they don't even want to have sex. Meanwhile, you have reached your peak and are as horny as a teenage boy!

The pregnancy details are fun to share. You are both excited and nervous at the same time. How exciting to hear the heartbeat and see the baby kick! I loved to play music for the baby, read to the baby, and watch the baby move. This was such a special time, and I wanted to share (and probably bore my husband to an extent) everything I could feel and see that was happening in order for us to become parents. One of my "party tricks" while I was pregnant was to get out my Doppler, which I used to hear the baby's heartbeat. I would place it just where I thought was the right place and let everyone hear the sweet little heartbeat of my unborn child. I had done this more times than I could count when someone told me that where I was placing the Doppler was just picking up on my own heartbeat. Oops, nobody else was the wiser. They all thought it was the baby, too!

Think I don't remember the freaky stuff that happened to my body during pregnancy? Oh I remember, but girl, you ain't seen nothing yet. What I'm talking about are the details of just what is going on with your body afterward. Here's the deal. . . You want your hubby/baby's daddy (I'll use these terms interchangeably, so use whatever applies to you best) to share the experience of pregnancy and childbirth, but you don't want to expose him to too much about your body. I didn't want my hubby to see me only as the mother of his kids and no longer his wife and lover after our children were born. Not sure about you, but I enjoy having sex with my husband and wanted to continue to have sex after I had kids! Guys are so visual and don't need to see just what is going on with you physically. They can be extremely supportive without getting details about bleeding, hemorrhoids, leaking, or any of the other fun things you experience. Spare them from having to overcome anything to continue to be attracted to their wife. They will see enough even if you aren't trying to throw it in their face.

We made a huge mistake in the delivery room with our first child. My husband has a very weak stomach. Right after the birth of our precious daughter, they brought her to my chest and then took her over to the bassinet. My husband walked over to the other side of the room to be with the baby. Then, he looked back at me, while adoring his new baby. *Big mistake!* Just because the baby is born doesn't mean the docs are done with you. It takes a little while in the delivery room until you are no longer spread eagle in all your birthing glory! Ryan always stayed by my head and saw our babies born, but he didn't need a front row seat! Well, he sure got an eyeful. The doctor works on the mom after the baby is born to get the afterbirth out, clean her, and sew her up if needed. We all thought he was going to pass out right there in the delivery room. I know I will never see that same look he had on his face again. Nobody but an OB/GYN needs to see all that! Especially not your husband! They don't need to ever try and get that picture out of their head!

Your hubbies have tremendous respect for you going through pregnancy, labor, and delivery. No matter how easy or rough the pregnancy has been on you, they are so relieved they aren't responsible for carrying and birthing a child. They don't have to see and be a part of every detail in order to know how much women have to go through. Spare your husband and help regain your sex life quicker. Trust me, you will want a sex life again one day! If your husband is in the delivery room, which he better be, then he has been exposed to enough!

Chapter 2

At the Hospital/ Girl Parts

Today's recordings come to you as I get ready to get in the shower. My five year old is at kindergarten, my twenty-two month old is in the highchair with fruit loops and a banana watching cartoons, and the baby is in his swing. I'm going to get in the shower and hope that I hear myself over the shower as I talk a little bit about what you need to know while you are at the hospital. Let me first start out by saying that all of my deliveries were very traditional hospital deliveries. I am intrigued by nontraditional labor methods and know that there are benefits to each type of delivery option available. Home births, water births, doulas, and lots of other alternative options are very interesting to me, but I went the traditional route. I couldn't imagine being anywhere but a hospital surrounded by nurses and doctors when it came time for childbirth. Most of this information will still work if you are in a home or different environment—I mean the first couple of days after delivery, for me, it was in the hospital.

Even though my deliveries were not at all what I would have planned, my overall hospital experience was very positive with all three of my children. I was induced each time, even though every time I initially planned on holding out for nature to take its course. I agreed with my docs each time induction was recommended due to three different reasons, but I still wonder what would have happened if I would have waited for me to go on my own. I never got to experience the middle of the night "my water just broke" excitement. I do wonder if my deliveries would have been easier if I wasn't induced, but no regrets. We were blessed with three amazing children, and I am grateful for the medical care we received in order to make that happen!

Just in case you are wondering what to pack to wear at the hospital and what to wear home from the hospital, it still needs to be maternity clothes! Maternity clothes or *really* loose elastic bottoms and loose tops. I have heard people joke about taking regular clothes. One of my friends at work said she was guilty of having done that, but I was a little more realistic. If you are not a first-time mom, then you completely understand this. If you are a first-time mom, let me explain. When you have your baby, you don't go right back down to your pre-pregnancy size! You will still look pregnant, feel pregnant (minus the little kickboxer in there), and need maternity clothes for a little while. You will have enough body issues going on; the last thing you need is clothes that are too tight. You sure don't need to be frustrated that you can't get your pants on. Now, I don't mean your one-size-too-big, bloated-day jeans in the closet, either. Not that they would button, but you would have to be able to pull them up over your hips in the first place. If you are like me, that's not happening anytime soon. Stick to elastic!

I always took the maternity clothes I was wearing at about six months pregnant to wear home and that worked well for me. You will be in your hospital gown most of the time the day you deliver, but I always took comfy pajamas to wear for visitors. Cotton jammies, with good coverage, work great for being in the hospital bed. Take several pairs, in case they get stained! Elastic-waist pajamas a size or two bigger than you would normally wear should work okay. They will just be stretched a little more in the hospital than when you are wearing them at home once you have lost some of your baby weight. You will be emotional enough that you don't need any additional heartache concerning clothes.

I would also take maternity underwear! Even if you didn't wear them during your pregnancy, buy some for the hospital! Two reasons: First, you will need some big-time granny panties to hold the huge pads you have on in place, and in the event of a C-section, they are comfortable. Let me explain. You will be bleeding a lot after you have your baby! You are going to want to wear the biggest pads you have ever worn, so you won't have to worry about saturating the pads while your family and friends are there visiting. The hospital will provide you with some complimentary giant pads, but bring some with you. I wanted to make sure there was no chance of leakage with people stopping in to see the baby (and see me, but really just the baby).

When I go visit my friends after giving birth, of course I want to see them and give them my love, but there is nothing more amazing than holding a newborn baby! I used to be so intimidated to hold new babies within days of their birth. I would hold them awkwardly afraid their head would fall off, and then give them back as soon as possible. Not anymore! Ever since I've had my own, there is absolutely nothing like it. So I completely get it when your visitors come in the room, make sure you are okay, and then spend the rest of the time all wrapped up in that sweet little bundle of joy.

Sorry, back to the gigantic pads that you will want. I would double up on pads, I mean, wear the crazy big hospital pads attached to your panties and then put the heavy flow ones that you brought on top. That's what I did, so there was no way I would leak through. Even if the top one got saturated, then the bottom one would just start soaking it up. If it hadn't leaked through to the bottom one, then I would just change the one on top and the bottom one would still be in place to continue to use.

If you have a C-section, you will really want some very high-waist maternity and/or granny panties. During my first pregnancy, I wore maternity panties only at the end of my pregnancy. With my other two pregnancies, I just wore my regular ones. They fit me a little differently than normal, but I got tired of having on huge panties all the time. So, with the third delivery, I had packed only regular panties. I should have brought granny panties no matter what to hold the jumbo pads I would be wearing, but I expected a vaginal delivery and didn't think about bringing anything else. When I ended up with a C-section, I didn't think I would bleed much anyway. Wrong, you will still bleed like crazy! Well, when I first put on panties, I made the mistake of using a regular pair. Ouch! Your C-section incision is very low and you won't want elastic anywhere close to it! The last thing you need is your undies irritating and rubbing your incision site. Maternity panties will be high enough that they won't bother your incision. So, no matter how your baby gets here, you will want giant panties to match your giant maxi pads!

You have the option while you are in the hospital of having your baby stay with you all night long or sending your baby to the nursery. I know you are so in love with this sweet, precious baby you have just been introduced to, but let your baby go to the nursery! You will have around the clock with this little baby soon enough, so while you can, rest! Love your baby, hold your baby, and feed your baby while your baby is in the room. Then as soon as they offer, send your baby on to the nursery. The nurses know what they are doing and will take great care of your baby. You need to heal and rest as much as you can before you go home and there's not a team of professional labor and delivery nurses waiting to take care of your child.

You will not have this luxury again, so take advantage while you can! You will still see your baby plenty, especially if you are breastfeeding. The nurses will bring your baby to you at least every three hours to nurse during the night. Your baby will be in good hands; get those small blocks of sleep while you can. You don't know just how much sleep you may be getting those first few nights when you bring the baby home. If it's like my first, the baby will have his or her days and nights completely backward. I knew this during my pregnancy. Every night when I went to bed, the dance party would begin. My first baby was most active during the night. As soon as I brought her home from the hospital, I realized it was because she was used to sleeping all day and being up most of the night!

Trust me; you won't regret sending your baby to the nursery while in the hospital!

The shower, I have to talk to you about the shower. I guess this is appropriate to talk about now, since I started this chapter while I was in the shower. *Your first shower is wonderful!* There is nothing like that first shower after you have had your baby. I, thankfully, have never been in a situation where I did not have the opportunity to bathe for a long period of time, but this is what finally getting a shower must feel like. The hospital is not the ideal place to take a shower, but it will be one of the best showers of your life! Let me tell you how good it feels. Just to stand in the warm water and get clean is amazing! And now, the shower has become my sanctuary. No kids have been allowed in with me since I had my baby, and it's the only little bit of alone time I get all day. *I feel clean,* and it feels great, if only for a few minutes. I'm still bleeding, and I smell like sour milk half the time because I've leaked through my nursing pads. When I'm in the shower, I am completely clean and fresh and you can't imagine how good it feels. So ladies, enjoy that first shower right after you give birth, and then continue to enjoy your shower sanctuary. I recommend taking advantage of a shower while your hubby is at home.

This way you aren't constantly listening for a crying baby or have your baby sitting in front of you the whole time.

My next piece of advice for the hospital, take the pain pills! You might as well while they are being offered. I have lots of respect for everyone who chooses to have a natural childbirth with no pain medication, and if that is what you are planning, then ignore the following advice. I chose an epidural with all three of my deliveries and never considered anything else. It didn't work very well with my first, and I felt far more than I would have liked. During the major contractions, while I was dilating to ten centimeters, it worked beautifully. This was an all-day process, and by the time I needed to push, I was able to move my legs completely and could feel everything—or at least I think I did. I had nothing to compare it to, but the doc was surprised that I could move my legs like normal. I put them up in stirrups with no trouble during labor, not at all the tree trunks my friends described. My doc was shocked that I could feel every contraction and knew just when to push. The extreme pain and pressure was overwhelming! My second delivery involved a much better epidural. I felt pressure but that was basically it, no extreme pain like my first.

Whether or not you choose to take the epidural, you also choose whether or not to take something for the pain following your delivery. I took it and am glad I did! It will make you feel better, and you need to be able to enjoy these first few days when you get to meet your sweet baby for the first time and share in the excitement with close friends and family. So take advantage of them, whatever they offer, whenever they offer them. They would give me something like ibuprofen every eight hours, but as for the good stuff, they don't keep them coming. They would be willing to give it to me every four hours, but wouldn't bring it to me again unless I asked for it. They don't keep up with when enough time has passed that you can take another dose. So I learned to keep pen and paper by me and kept track of when medication was last given. You don't want to wait until you realize you haven't had it long after it's due because you are hurting! It's much harder to get pain under control than it is to keep it under control, so stay on top of it and ask for more when it's time.

Now, don't peg me as a pill popper! I very rarely even take ibuprofen or acetaminophen at home. I do not like having medicine head and have to be in pretty bad shape before I will take any pain reliever. But after childbirth, that is different! If you've had surgery with a C-section or a traumatic vaginal delivery, then it is justified! I know there are exceptions to every rule, and some new moms may truly not need it. I still have a very vivid memory of the pain, and I recall that I needed something regularly for pain! You also don't have to worry about the safety of your baby. The labor and delivery departments would never give you anything that would harm your baby through breast milk. Think of being preventative with your pain management instead of waiting until it is too late.

In the hospital, you are so overwhelmed with the fact that you just had a baby and just experienced this miracle that you aren't concentrating on yourself, but more the baby. So I can say that even though my births weren't easy, I actually felt good with proper pain management while in the hospital. With my vaginal births, I was up walking and hanging out with friends enjoying their company and celebrating the day after I had delivered. Between the medicine and the high of meeting your child for the first time, that first day or two in the hospital wasn't too bad. I was sore, but not at all what I expected. Once those painkillers stop coming and you are probably doing more than you should, reality sets in and you hurt. After my first vaginal delivery, my "stuff" was *so sore*! The first week home I hurt; I hurt really bad.

Now is the time I need to decide how I am going to reference the female genitalia. I am struggling with this a little bit because I don't want to be crude. I'm thinking I will use the same terms that my five-year-old daughter and I use. We call the female genitalia *girl parts*. I know all the experts say to use proper medical terminology with your children, but I can't bring myself to do it. When they are older, I will inform them of all the proper names, but for now, no way I'm saying *vagina* around my five-year-old daughter. We use the terms *tatas* or *boobs* when talking about breasts, so I will do the same.

With our first, we weren't sure when it was no longer appropriate for our daughter to see her dad naked. Ryan and I were so used to it just being the two of us that we hadn't thought much about having our first baby around when we were changing clothes or in the shower. Even after our second was born, we just always let our kids come and go from the bathroom when one of us was in the shower. We have a tile shower with a glass door and mostly glass sides, so if you are in the bathroom you can see right into whoever is in the shower. There is no privacy if anyone else is in the bathroom with you. We used to never lock the door. Lots of times, I take a shower with my baby in a bouncy seat right in front of me, and his big sisters are running in and out of the bathroom. Now, we feel we have to pay a little more attention when Ryan is taking a shower and make sure he's not naked as a jaybird around our girls anymore.

I feel very strongly that my girls are comfortable seeing me naked. I remember being in grade school, and my friend told me that her sister had hair "down there." I thought she was crazy and didn't know what she was talking about. That was the grossest thing I had ever heard. I soon figured out that it was the norm and not some kind of abnormality! I had a big sister, too, but we were very modest around our house. I don't remember seeing my mom or sister naked. I know my sister and I took baths together when we were little, but as we got older we never saw each other naked. I think it's a generational thing because I've had this discussion with friends and they have similar situations.

I want my girls to know what a mature woman's body looks like. I'm glad they have a little brother, too, so they know how a boy is different from a girl. They are very intrigued with his little parts. At first, my oldest and her girl cousins didn't miss a diaper change out of sheer curiosity. I don't mind at all while he's a baby, and I'm glad they will already know what makes us different and hopefully not go looking for the answers and pictures themselves. Our girls, however, don't need to know what a mature male looks like at this point, especially their dad! Not only did our girls come and go as we were in the shower, but half the time they wanted to get in, too. As long as we weren't in a hurry, both Ryan and I would let them. They love our big shower and thought it was so much fun to take one with mom or dad. That is, until our oldest made *the comment.*

She was about three years old when we decided the door needed to be locked when daddy was in the shower because she started paying way too much attention to his genitals. One day, she was in the shower with her dad, and when she got out, she came over to me and said, "Mommy, Daddy has *really big* girl parts!" So, no more daddy showers. It was obvious she was no longer oblivious! We explained that he didn't have girl parts, but he had *boy parts* and left it at that. If you ever wonder if it's time for your children to no longer see a parent of the opposite sex naked, have no fear. The child will eventually say something to let you know it's time to be much more discreet! Now, Ryan took it as a compliment, as any man would. I thought it was hilarious! Recently, while my oldest was watching me change our son's diaper, she said, "It kind of looks like a hotdog." I just let that go, and I haven't heard any more comments about boy parts since, but I'm sure there will be so many more questions to come.

Back to your girl parts. After you are no longer on pain meds and you are down from the happy cloud of just becoming a mom, *get ready.* Sorry to have to tell you this. *It hurts!* You expect yourself to hurt because you just gave birth. You just pushed a baby out of a very small opening, or at least what used to be a very small opening. But I could have never expected this! It is so sore; just to sit down or try and get comfortable enough to lie down is not easy. I had to have an episiotomy with both my vaginal births. An episiotomy is where they have to cut you in order to get the baby out without you ripping beyond repair. And surprisingly, my first vaginal delivery with my 8-pounder was a much harder recovery than my second vaginal delivery with my 11-pound little girl, or I guess I should say big girl. I think that is just the difference between my first and second baby. That area was undisturbed before my first and took longer to recover from the trauma of a first-time delivery! So, at least for me, my first vaginal recovery was much harder and longer than my second.

When you are in the hospital and you have to go to the bathroom for the first time after childbirth, let me warn you, it is not pleasant! For quite some time after I had vaginal deliveries, I had to rise up from the toilet out of pain trying to manage what was happening to me, just to pee! It doesn't last that long, but it is awful! Get ready for the first time you have to poop, too! (We will use the same five year old terms for this.) When you have to poop, oh my gosh, it hurts really bad! They will offer stool softeners, and you need to take them and keep taking them long after you get home. Take them as long as you need to. Right now, a month after my C-section, I am still taking stool softeners. You don't want to stress with trying to push while going to the bathroom when you are sore at the sight from a vaginal delivery or so sore from your incision with a C-section.

While your girl parts are this sore, I also recommend using sitz baths and tucks pads. After my first vaginal delivery, I would do sitz baths all the time. There was nothing that felt better or gave me more relief than a sitz bath. A sitz bath is a fountain for your coochie. I can't believe I just said coochie—you know what I mean, girl parts! Hope that doesn't offend anyone! It's going to be a long time before my girls are reading this, so I guess I don't have to stick with only five- year-old terms, but I still can't bring myself to say vagina all the time. The sitz bath is a fountain of warm water or water and witch hazel that shoots up all over that area. It doesn't sound that impressive, but at the time, it feels wonderful! I didn't use them much with my second delivery, but I *loved* them with my first delivery. You may not want to go to the trouble of actually using the apparatus of a sitz bath. (It's a plastic tub that sits over the toilet that has a hose connected to it. You fill it with water and then the water shoots out of it.) You can also just use a plastic squirt bottle. They gave me one in the hospital, but a plastic ketchup dispenser will work just fine. You just fill it up with water or a combo of water and witch hazel and spray it where you want!

Also, get some witch hazel pads, like Tucks. You will love these, too! They work great for a lot of reasons. You are not going to feel clean for a long time after you have your baby because you are leaking and bleeding, so this works great for hygiene to clean yourself when you go to the bathroom. They are also very soothing. What I did for a long time was put several in my panties over my pad. They are about the size of a peanut butter lid. Just take several and line them up on your pad. Leave them so they are up against you and replace as often as necessary. This will give you some relief, but there is absolutely no preparing you completely for your first few bathroom experiences after delivery. It was very rough, but like all the things you will deal with during this time, it doesn't last very long.

After my first episiotomy, I felt like I had been ripped open! I remember getting out a mirror to try and see what it looked like and if everything was where it was supposed to be. I just felt like I had been ripped from one side to the other. Everything was as it should be; they sewed me up where I needed to be sewn, but it sure didn't feel like it! You will also feel and look very swollen down there. You swell down there during your pregnancy, so you are used to it a little, but it is even more exaggerated right after delivery. Everything will return to normal, I promise, but you don't think it's possible when you are feeling like this. You will bleed for a long time too. Your uterus is contracting to shrink back to the size it was before pregnancy. As the lining of your uterus sheds, you will bleed like you are on a very heavy period. So just wear a heavy pad all the time so you don't worry about spotting.

Chapter 3
C-section and Vaginal Deliveries

With a C-section, I didn't have sore girl parts. That was great! I'm not going to say that one was necessarily better or easier than the other because there are advantages to both. You are the same amount of woman no matter how you deliver your baby. If you are determined to have a vaginal birth, but the doctors decide a C-section is safe, don't sweat it. As long as you and your baby make it through childbirth safely, it was a success! I will tell you that one major advantage to a C-section is no trauma to your girl parts! You will be very sore from where the incision is, of course, but things are so much easier downstairs! It didn't hurt like hell to sit down or pee, and that was such a relief after having gone through vaginal births twice before. Also, I'm guessing the first time you have sex again isn't so scary! More info to come on that subject!

You do have a longer recovery with a C-section because you have just had major surgery and your body needs to heal. You have to take it easy to make sure that your incision closes properly, but the pain of the incision site is really the only thing that hurts. Even that wasn't as bad as I expected. I do know people who were fully dilated before a C-section was called, and they had the soreness of girl parts along with the incision site. So thankful I only had to deal with one of these issues at a time. I was very surprised after my C-section because I didn't have to do anything to the actual incision site. I was expecting to have to do wound care, but there wasn't any. What my doctor gave me wasn't even staples; it was just glue. There were internal stitches that didn't have to be removed; they just dissolved. The glue just flakes away in time, so I could even take showers like normal right afterward.

You need to follow the medical advice you are given about limiting your activity and not picking up anything heavy. You will be tempted to hoist the stroller in the car, carry the baby around in the car seat, and so many other things. Don't do it! These restrictions are given for a reason. Even if you feel good and your incision looks to be healing well, you could do major damage and have a huge setback in your recovery. If you overdo it, you could risk pulling your stitches out. I've heard way too many horror stories about complications after a C-section. Lord knows you don't need to add any self-inflicted troubles after having a baby, so don't push it!

With a vaginal delivery, you are much more sore at home than you were at the hospital. You are up and moving around your house, not on as much pain medication, and you are trying to function in your home with a new baby. Coming home from a hospital stay and being very sore from whatever procedure you just had takes some patience and recovery time. Throw a brand new baby who needs you around the clock into the mix, and it doesn't leave much time for you to concentrate on your healing process.

Continue to regularly take the pain pills that you were prescribed upon discharge. You will still want to wear your pads around the clock because the bleeding will last much longer, but it shouldn't hurt quite as bad to pee at this point.

For me, it turned from hurting at my girl parts to throbbing. This weird uncomfortable throbbing feeling right at your girl parts is hard to describe. I know I could feel my heart beating at my coochie at one point! I don't know why this happens, but it is a very strange, aching, unpleasant feeling that you can't get off your mind. It's kind of hard to have a conversation with someone or really concentrate on anything else when you have this constant pressure and throbbing happening down there. Of course, you are still very swollen, and it feels like you are never going to get back what you used to recognize as your girl parts, but you will! It's all for a short time, but it feels like it will never return to normal when you are feeling and looking like this! You won't always be swollen five times the size you were before baby down there. Going to the bathroom will continue to get a little easier, but the soreness will get worse. Just make it as comfortable for yourself as possible. Use lots of pillows to sit on and don't forget to place the tucks pads in your panties!

I was swollen everywhere with a C-section! My entire body blew up right afterward! I don't know if it was the C-section or surgery in general, but it was awful! I never reacted like this going through all my pregnancies. I swelled the most with my first pregnancy, but hardly swelled any with my second and third pregnancy. Swelling during pregnancy was nothing like right after the surgery, I was huge! With my first baby, I was given a pedicure just a little before I was going to deliver. The lady doing my nails said she had worked on several other pregnant ladies in the same week. I told her she must have been used to working on swollen feet then, and she said, "No, not really, your feet are much bigger." Thanks lady, as if I didn't already have a complex about my monster feet that I didn't even recognize anymore. They were squares—big cinderblocks at the end of my legs. Good thing I couldn't see them very easily! But nothing compared to the swelling after my C-section. You should have seen my cankles at this point! My feet, my legs, my stomach, I was swollen everywhere! When I asked if I should be concerned in the hospital, they said that was just a side effect to having the surgery, but I am warning you to be ready for this! I had no idea that could happen.

Also, where you have your incision feels foreign and so strange. Right there where they cut you open feels weird. For me, the best way to describe it is like a jellyfish sitting on your lower abdomen. There is very little feeling there, and it stands away from your body and feels like it's almost on top of your skin. It is this squishy mass laying on top of your skin that is stuck to you. Even now it feels like that a little bit. Not at all like the first couple of weeks, but it's still this foreign mushy area that I hope will feel like a part of me at some point. I'm now a month out from my C-section. It's still an unrecognizable blob that doesn't belong, but at least it's a smaller blob than it was a few weeks ago. Some people have told me I will never get feeling back in that area completely, but who cares if I am a little numb down at my bikini line. As long as this extra floppy area goes away, I will be okay.

I am nervous about what it is going to look like. I don't think of myself as a superficial person, but I wonder if it will always look strange. I don't know what the scar will look like in time; I don't know if it will ever get flat again. There is a place just above where the incision was that bulges over. I wonder if it's even possible to tighten that area up with exercise or if there will always be an extra flap of skin. Either way, it was worth it! My pole dancing days are behind me anyway! Ha ha! And remember, maternity panties are still necessary at this point. I know I talked about wanting them at the hospital, but you are going to want them for a long time once you get home. The incision site is sore, and no matter how they put you back together, you won't want to irritate it by having a waistband rub on it. That glue stuff starts to peel off, and I definitely don't want the elastic from my panties rubbing it. So, if you know you are having a C-section, I would stock up on granny panties if you weren't already wearing them before you had your baby.

What else about a C-section surprised me? Gas! The nurse came in my hospital room and said, "Are you having much gas?" At that point I wasn't. I said, "No, not really." I kind of wondered why she was asking. Well, it didn't take long to figure it out! I think just her asking the question made it all kick in! I was so gassy! This is one of those things that my husband was a part of because you can't really hide it. I would be lying there in the bed watching TV, and this air would just come through me and make the loudest noises I have ever heard come out of me. Apparently, this is supposed to happen, but it's still so embarrassing. My hospital room was right outside of the nurses' station, and I could have sworn that everyone at that nurses' station heard me passing gas. So C-section ladies, be ready for crazy loud gas, big-time bloating, and the foreign jellyfish thing that becomes a part of your lower abdomen. I'm glad to say I haven't had explosive gas now in quite some time, and my jellyfish has shrunk incredibly! Now, I know all this doesn't sound very appealing, but at least your girl parts won't be in shambles!

When you get home, be ready to bleed after a C-section just like you do with a vaginal delivery. I don't know why I thought it would be so different. I guess I just thought they clean everything out when they operate. Either way, you are still shedding the uterine lining, and lots of blood is to be expected. I bled like a heavy period leading into about two weeks, and then it lightened up. I had a scare at this point. The biggest blood clot came even after I wasn't bleeding so heavy anymore. Out of the blue, when I was going to the bathroom, I shed a huge blood clot. It was unlike any bleeding I have done with my vaginal births. Good thing I was on the toilet,
because if it would have happened in my pad, I know I would have freaked out even more. It scared me, so I started researching and talking to others and found out that was not uncommon at all.

My hospital told us that if you fill up a pad in less than an hour or pass a clot larger than a half dollar to call your doctor. Two weeks out, I didn't think anything like this would happen. Thank goodness I was just hanging out at home with Ryan and the kids when it did happen. I had a letdown that felt like what I would expect your water breaking would feel like, and that's when I ran to the bathroom. My pad was saturated and blood just poured out of me, and then it was done. I got to the living room and felt it again, so I ran back to the bathroom, and that's when I passed the crazy big clot. It was a very weird sensation, then I went back to light bleeding. It all happened over about a thirty-minute period, then all was normal. No crazy trip to the ER or anything because I was right back to normal, but don't hesitate to call your doctor or seek medical attention with excessive bleeding. That was on a Sunday, then a few days later, I had a mini-version of it again when I was out and about running errands. Nothing like the first clot, though, and ever since I have been bleeding very little. So here's what to expect from my experience . . . heavy bleeding first couple of weeks, passed clots over a few days, then very light bleeding at a month out. With my vaginal deliveries, it varied a little bit how long and how heavy I bled. I never had a time where I passed that large of a clot. I had lots of little clots in the weeks after I had given birth, but nothing as extreme as the one after the C-section.

I am trying to be realistic and I have come to the conclusion that this book is not going to happen by the end of the summer. That's okay because I am loving this! This book has become my vice, or as my husband calls it my "crack." Once I start, I can't stop. I love working on getting all these recordings down on paper. I am now awake most nights when he gets home around 11:30 pm. I start writing as soon as the kids are all in bed and am bright-eyed and wired when he walks through the door. It used to be that I would be sound asleep or trying to keep my eyes open watching TV or reading a book. Now, late night is my time to write, and I am so sad that I will have to give it up. The start of the school year is fast approaching, and with that we have to get back on our school schedule. This means I have to get up early every morning once again. Even on the days I'm off work, I have to leave the house before 7:00 am to get my oldest to school on time.

I know I need my sleep, and I can't keep staying up to the middle of the night, so this will become my Monday book. On Mondays I am off work, and with our new schedule, I will have only one child at home, my youngest. My middle child just started preschool four days a week. When you have one child, it's hard to accomplish anything while he or she is awake. Now with three, give me one kid at the house, and I can get all kinds of stuff done. I am looking forward to having one-on-one time with my youngest, but while he is occupied and asleep, I plan on getting more of this book written. I am not going to give myself any deadline at this point. It will be finished when I am finished. I know I'm going to have to clean my house on my Mondays when it's completed, so I'm not in a big hurry.

Chapter 4
Accept Help

I'm going to give some advice that I am really bad about taking myself. After you have had your baby, whenever anyone offers to do anything for you, take them up on it! You need your rest. You never know how much sleep you are going to be getting at night. Nobody has to stay around the clock. I love my extended family, but I didn't want them at my house all night long. It's such a special time for your immediate family to share in welcoming a baby into your home, and I just don't like somebody else in my house constantly. If you want others to spend the night, and they are willing and able, then let them. For me, a few hours during the day was perfect. Whether it is coming over to stay with you a little bit or taking things off the to-do list, let them help! Just don't shun people away when they offer. You may think you have it all covered, and you can do it all by yourself, but there is no better time to use a support system of friends and family than now. If someone just stops by and does the dishes, *wow*! If somebody is able to come over and fold a couple loads of laundry, *wonderful*! If someone holds and feeds the baby if you aren't breastfeeding to give you a couple hours to take a nap, *sweet*! Everyone always says sleep when the baby sleeps. Great advice, but nothing else will ever get done. I always did that during the night, but seldom during the day. I can't just go take a nap when I have a chance to do a few things that don't involve this sweet little baby!

Hopefully, your husband/baby's daddy will be home with you a little while after the baby is born. Most are able to take at least a couple days off work when you get home, maybe a week. It seems like the more kids you have, the less time your husband feels is necessary to be off work to help out. You really don't need him as much as you do that first time. By your second baby, you're not wondering if your motherly instinct is ever going to kick in or worried that something will happen to your baby if you are not holding him or her every second. When you have that first baby, a week off is usually the norm. Some new dads are even home for weeks after the baby is born. Then you have your third kid, and he's like, "You're being induced on Thursday, great. I'll just take a long weekend and go back to work on Monday." You've got the baby thing down, but now you have several kids you are trying to balance. It is easier because you're not so nervous about your newborn, but there are so many more demands with several kids of different ages and stages. This is when you need all the help you can get.

Dinners are the best! Several of my friends and family members brought meals to the house and even stocked up my fridge and freezer with quick meals. I'm not one who enjoys cooking that much anyway, so it was fantastic! I have a wonderful support system, and my extended family has been so good to help make everything happen. When I had my first child, my mom, mother-in-law, and sister came over and helped me get used to this crazy, wonderful new role of motherhood. What I needed most then was wisdom from them on not being so nervous about having a newborn baby and help trying to figure out just what to do.

When it came to my second and third babies, they all helped out so much with our existing children. You have to have someone with them while your hubby is with you during the hospital stay. I think it's best to keep the older children on as regular of a schedule as possible, so someone needs to take them to and from school and to the hospital to visit. Ryan didn't stay in the hospital with me the entire time I was there, and he didn't stay all day while my youngest was still in the NICU. So it was a combination of him and family getting the siblings where they needed to be. If nobody offers to do something specific that you need, just ask for it! This is one of those times when it is impossible for you and your baby's daddy to be everywhere you need to be when necessary. I'm guilty of wanting to do everything myself, but I had to let it go! Somebody else can pick out what your kids wear for a week and help with homework. Trust me, you will have plenty of time to do all that with them before you know it.

Let me also warn you if you have older children that there is a good possibility a guilt trip is coming your way.

You will not be able to attend something, take them to school, or do something they expect only you to do with them. The normal routine is going to be disrupted for a little while; there is no way around it! This time, our schedule was interrupted longer than expected because of staying in the hospital for so many days with my C-section and having to keep our baby in the NICU even longer. The week after my baby finally got to come home from the hospital, my five year old had her first kindergarten field trip. He was only two weeks old, and we had only had him home for one week. I walked her into school that morning like normal. She knew she had a field trip that day and was excited about it. In the front of the lobby stood all of the parents going on the field trip because they were leaving early that morning. I walked her to the set of double doors that lead to her classroom hallway, like always, and she asks, “Why are all those parents back there?” I didn’t think twice and I told her they were going on the field trip with them. She looked at them and back at me and completely lost it! She was crying hysterically! Huge tears were running down her cheeks while she was asking, “Why aren’t you going? I want you to go on the field trip with me.”

Okay, I'm two weeks after a C-section. I am not going to be chasing a bunch of five year olds around the pumpkin patch. Even if I felt up to it, no way I was leaving this baby boy for a second—definitely not for an entire day! So I have her clinging to me with big tears running down her cheeks. One of the teachers comes over and pries her off my leg and gets her to walk with her on down to her classroom. I go up to my friends and explain what is going on while I am trying my best to keep it together. I go get in my car and cry all the way home. Don't know how long she was emotional, but I sure didn't get over it very quick. Those sweet mommas sent me updates and pictures all morning. My girl was loving every minute of the pumpkin patch with a huge smile on her face, even without her mom there! I guess it's a good thing. Now that we have three children, I don't need to have my oldest think that I will be able to be there for absolutely everything, although I have been up until this point. I do now have to divide my time among three kids and my part-time job. I can't always continue to volunteer and be at every school function that comes along. She isn't quite ready for the fact that mommy can't be at absolutely everything all the time.

Chapter 5 Hemorrhoids – A Pain in the Ass

Here's another one of those fun things I never shared with my husband. Hemorrhoids. I remember my first job out of college when one of the girls I worked with had just come back from maternity leave. She complained about hemorrhoids all the time, and I thought she was bonkers. None of my close friends or my sister had become moms yet. I had no clue or care about pregnancy and having babies at the time. I knew what hemorrhoids were, but I had no idea they were a side effect of labor and delivery and that so many new mommas experienced them. Honestly, at the time, I didn't care and thought she was obnoxious about giving random personal details to a bunch of women at work. She was very descriptive, and I remember her comparing them to grapes attached to your butt crack. *What in the world?* Well, I can relate now. She told only a few ladies at work what she was going through. What a difference a few years make!

> Thank goodness for spellcheck; that's one of the hardest words ever to spell. Imagine that in a spelling bee. When they ask for a definition, I can see it now. "Hemorrhoids—those blood blisters in your ass that hurt like hell after having a baby!" Need it used in a sentence, okay. "I hate having hemorrhoids right now because it makes me think I am dying every time I have to poop!"

Now I'm going to try to get this book published with all my personal issues out there for everybody to know.

If you don't know what hemorrhoids are, let me clue you in. Hemorrhoids are swollen veins, like little pockets of blood that are in your crack and are very uncomfortable! I get why she compared them to grapes, but mine were not near that big, and thank God I didn't have a cluster of them. It doesn't matter if you have one or several or how big they are, you can bet that they will be an actual pain in your ass! You already have your girl part issues; why do you have to have something going on back there, too? They bleed and hurt, then go away and pop back up so randomly. When you are pushing and straining during labor, there's a good chance hemorrhoids are in your future. I guess you may be able to spare them with scheduled C-sections, but I was lucky enough to get them each and every time. I have been told that they never truly disappear; it's just a matter of whether or not they flare up. You would never know you have them when they aren't swollen, but they really hurt when they are acting up. It's uncomfortable all the time, and when you have to poop, it is ridiculously painful. You would think they would pop up immediately after going through labor. For me, it was always a few weeks after the fact.

So, if you have blood in your stool after delivery and it hurts like hell, it's probably a hemorrhoid. Congrats, one more joy of motherhood! There are all kinds of creams you can buy to shrink them. You can use those same Tucks witch hazel pads you use for your girl parts to relieve hemorrhoids, too; they work great to soothe them. You can even leave them a little farther back in your panties to help get relief back there.

I don't really understand why I am dealing with them right now after having a C-section. I never even pushed! I never dilated beyond 5 centimeters, but here they are, once again! They even came back a little bit during this pregnancy, which I don't get, either. Here's another reason for stool softeners. As long as you have them flaring up, take stool softeners! This will make so much difference in how painful it is when you have to go to the bathroom! You may want to get your ketchup/squirt bottle back out again, too. Sitz baths or warm water will feel great for hemorrhoids. Just aim a little farther back this time! And, please spare your husbands. You can vent to him that you are dealing with them, but no need to give details! If my hubby reads this book, he's going to know all my troubles. Hopefully by the time that happens, I will be way past all these "oh so sexy" labor and delivery issues.

Chapter 6

Boobs Gone Wild

I'm on my way to the school to pick up my five year old. I'm early, so with drive time and car line, I should have some time to get some more thoughts down. Now is as good a time as any to start talking about boobs. I could probably write five chapters on just your tatas. Think you've seen some changes during pregnancy, that's nothing compared to what is to come! When you are in the hospital, it's another one of those things that isn't that bad. Your milk hasn't come in yet or has just started to, so they aren't out of control. When you get home, you will soon find out whether or not you will have enough milk to nurse (if that's what you want to do). I am a big supporter of nursing. Well, let me rephrase that. I'm very big on giving your child colostrum and breast milk. Whether they get it direct from the source or they get it from a bottle, who cares. Whatever works for you!

If you don't know about colostrum yet, it's what is first discharged from your nipples before your milk comes in. It's a thick, clear substance with a hint of yellow that is supposed to be jam packed with good stuff for your baby. If your milk comes in and you are able to nurse for any amount of time, then I would. It doesn't matter if it is two weeks or a year. My girls had only breast milk up until three months. Then, when I went back to work, I did a combination of breast milk and formula. I eventually weaned myself back where I had to pump or nurse only first thing in the morning and last thing at night.

So many people have very strong opinions on this! Do what works for you and your baby! I was a formula-fed baby. That's just what you did when my mom had kids.

Lots of my friends have done formula because enough milk didn't come in or that was just their preference. Yes, it's healthy to get all these nutrients and antibodies into your child through breast milk, but it's not worth stressing yourself out if it's not for you. I recommend at least trying it; you can always switch to formula at any time. Breastfeeding is a very strange experience. It is very awkward to have a baby attached to you. It was for me anyway.

You will find out very quickly how easy it is for your milk to come in. If you are like me with my first, my body was ready even before the baby arrived. I was leaking breast milk during the pregnancy. I didn't even think that was possible! The first time is so easy for me to remember because of where I was. Maybe stress brought it on, but I was only five months pregnant! My dad was having open heart surgery and I was at the hospital. My mom, sister, and I all stayed together the night before so we would be there bright and early for when they took dad to surgery. All of a sudden, I felt something weird. I looked down and there was a big pancake size wet spot on my shirt! Just know that you can leak before you even have your baby. If you're like me, it's a good sign that you won't have any problems with your milk coming in! Just wear the bra pads if this is happening, so you won't be caught in an extremely embarrassing moment!

The nurses at the hospital said milk is supposed to come in a couple days after a vaginal birth or about five days after a C-section. Mine came in very quickly with both types of deliveries. I never had any problems with that. Your boobs will be the biggest they have ever been. They are also warm, milk filled, and veiny. So they may be huge, but not attractive! Nice to have big cleavage, but I would rather have my pre-baby boobs any day. They look like big, milky mom tatas now. Definitely not big sexy boobs! During pregnancy, my boobs get bigger; when nursing, my boobs get huge. It's such a tease! I see the potential that could be there, if my boobs were only normal when they were that size. If they weren't mom boobs, but sexy boobs, that would be great! Then, right after I'm finished nursing, there they go. They deflate and it seems like they deflate even smaller each time. Who knows, maybe this is the time my boobs are here to stay! I'm not counting on it, but first time with a boy and we all know how boys like big boobs!

It's a strange sensation when your milk comes in. If you are going to nurse, then you will start trying to nurse before your milk is actually there. I've had a wonderful experience and also a terrible experience with nursing, so I can speak from both perspectives. Everybody talks about what an amazing bonding experience it is to breastfeed. I did not get that at all with my first child. It hurt; it was uncomfortable and very odd. Neither one of us knew what we were doing; it wasn't pleasant. I would cringe every time I thought about it being time for her to latch on. Even though it is supposed to be such a natural thing, it was so unnatural for me. She wouldn't latch on well, and when she finally did it was always in the wrong place. If they don't put their mouth directly over your nipple, it hurts! If she was anywhere close, and I thought she was getting some milk, then I would suffer through it. It felt like shards of glass being poked through my nipple.

I will never forget her first Easter. She was born early April, and to this point (only a couple weeks) I had only breastfed. She was screaming uncontrollably on Easter morning. My husband and I went to my parents' house for an Easter meal with her still screaming crying. My mom was worried she was hungry. I thought that wasn't the case, because it felt like I was nursing constantly. We put some formula in a bottle and gave it to her, and she ate like she was starving! I don't care how much or how long she was latching on, she obviously wasn't getting enough. So, from that point on, I started pumping. I would still try and nurse every once in a while, especially in the middle of the night. I didn't want to have to get up and take the time to pump and then feed her, but nursing always hurt. We never figured it out! Before long, I went to just pumping. I would pump whenever it was time for her to eat and then turn right around and give her the milk in a bottle. So that's what I did to get her breast milk. Once I was producing more milk, I would always stay at least one feeding ahead of her. I could feed her when she was hungry and then pump afterward and have one ready to go. At three months, I started doing a combo of breastmilk and formula so I didn't have to pump around the clock.

With my second child, we got it. The nursing thing worked! My little girl latched on beautifully. It was sweet. It was easy. I would rub her little head and cheeks while she was nursing, and it was a wonderful bonding experience. I don't know if it was me being nervous the first time or if my second child could just do it better. With my youngest it was a little different. With him having to stay in the NICU for a little while, I didn't get a chance to nurse initially. When he was ready to breastfeed in the NICU, it was the most amazing bonding experience ever! I had hardly gotten to hold my baby much up to that point.

So, when I was able to rock him and hold him to my chest, I felt like I was finally able to take care of him for the first time! It was and always will be one of my most sweet unforgettable mom moments. Then he got thrush. This is a yeast infection in a baby's mouth. The nurses explained what it would be like if he nursed during this time and that it would be passed onto me. Well, that weirded me out, so I decided to wait until it was gone before we nursed again. By the time it cleared up, he wouldn't latch on. He was used to the bottle, which was lots easier than getting milk out of my nipple, so it was back to pumping.

This time I pump like a professional. I can pump six ounces in three minutes with no problem. I have a large supply, and it's no hassle to pump because it's so quick. I used to just do one boob at a time and the other would be leaking everywhere as I was pumping. Now, two at once is no problem. It just looks a little awkward! Let me explain a few tips to keep you from getting engorged or mastitis, which is no fun! I had no idea your tatas were capable of hurting that bad! Your boobs feel like concrete when engorged and can quickly turn into infection. Do everything you can to prevent it! When your milk first comes in, you will feel a very warm sensation. If you nurse, then they say to do it ten to fifteen minutes on each side.

This sucking action will help promote your breast milk to continue to produce an adequate amount for what your baby needs. While you are in the hospital, the lactation specialists are there to help. They will help you figure out the most comfortable way to hold the baby and help make sure the baby is latched on properly.

If you only nurse, then you should produce just what your baby needs. Every time your baby is latched on, it is telling your body to produce more, more, more—the baby is still hungry. So don't use your boob as a pacifier. It's so easy to do when you are nursing. The baby is content, and you are able to relax (as long as it's a good nursing experience). Because of this, you are tempted to just rock the baby in that position, even nod off and take a little breather. The problem is, your boobs are being told this baby needs more milk and will go on overdrive because of that, and soon you will have more than enough, which leads to engorgement. When this happens your breasts become very tender and very sore. They are like a huge inflated balloon maxed out to how much it can hold. Trying to get your baby to latch on when your breasts are that inflated is not easy. Babies' mouths just slide right off and can't get hold of anything. They need soft skin to hold onto something, not just a hard rock with a nipple sticking out.

This is when you need to release a little milk prior to nursing. You can get in the shower and squirt some out. Warm water gets your milk flowing well. Most of my showers turn into milk baths! What worked best for me was to stand over the sink and express just a little out. It feels good to relieve some of the pressure, but don't overdo it. As soon as you empty them too much and then feed your baby, your body thinks it needs to start making more, and mastitis here we come! Get rid of just enough that your boobs are not completely full and the baby can latch on. I always had an abundance of milk, but if you don't it's like liquid gold. If you are at this point of engorgement, you have plenty too. If it took a long time to build up to this point, I know it's hard just to see it go down the drain. You can always squirt milk into a sterilized container, so you can use it later. You shouldn't be releasing much, though. It shouldn't even add up to an ounce.

My sister gave me great advice on this and showed me what to do. She had already experienced mastitis and was trying to prevent me from the same torture. I got painfully engorged at different times, but never had to be treated for mastitis! Engorgement is rock hard, very full boobs. Mastitis is an actual infection that needs to be treated with antibiotics. You should feel other symptoms like you would with any other infection and need to see your doctor. Your boobs will be tender and sore when you first start to breastfeed. There are a couple of things that will give you some relief when you are nursing. Warm showers are great, but heat makes you produce more milk. I have been told to take a warm shower if you are trying to get your milk to come in and make sure your back is to the warm water if you want it to dry up. This means that if you use a warm compress to relieve the soreness you may also be helping increase your production. I need relief the most when I am engorged, and the last thing I want to do is encourage more milk.

Cold packs felt so good when I was dealing with engorgement. You won't want to keep ice directly on your boobs, but cool packs feel great. I have been using Capri Sun packs this time. I wish I would have thought of it sooner. They work perfect and feel so good! One night I woke up and was dealing with the pain of engorgement just on one side. It was bad enough that I couldn't get back to sleep. I went to the freezer trying to figure out what I could use to give me some relief. Rock hard frozen ice packs or frozen corn didn't seem so appealing. I looked in the fridge and saw my kids' Capri Suns. I think everyone knows what these are, but just in case you don't, they are those drink pouches for kids. I tucked one under my shirt and it felt wonderful! You can always use the gel ice packs, which aren't so hard, but cold Capri Sun pouches work great for me. Just don't use too much ice because that is also recommended to dry up your milk. A little cool Capri Sun won't hurt your milk flow. Just remember heat produces more and cold helps stop your milk.

If everything works correctly, in time, nursing shouldn't hurt. I think the more kids you breastfeed, the tougher your nipples get too. My nipples were extremely sore with my first, and even though it was a good experience with my second, they were still sore. It was painful the moment that she latched on, then no problem once she started nursing. My nipples would get cracked and bleed. Sometimes when I pumped there would be a pink tint to the milk because of blood; it sure wasn't strawberry. I used a lot of lanolin cream to try and keep them from cracking. I highly recommend lanolin cream if you have the same trouble. I haven't had that issue at all this time, and the little bit I breastfed didn't hurt. But he doesn't want my boob anymore, so the decision to stop breastfeeding was made for me. This was probably the one time I would have had absolutely no pain breastfeeding. That's okay. I've got this pumping thing down. Thank you sister and sister-in-law for my pumps. I now have one set up at home and one for on the go!

Chapter 7

Pumping

At the moment I am doing laundry. My baby is taking a nap, and my toddler is watching cartoons. Let's see how much I can record while I fold laundry. Let me give you the basics on using a pump. You never imagine yourself needing or wanting to milk yourself, but that is exactly what you are doing. Initially, it is extremely awkward, but it will get to be not that big of a deal. Your nipple gets sucked into a cone and milk is pulled from it. The milk drops into the attached container, and *voila*, your baby's dinner is ready!

It's a negative pressure suction that imitates the baby sucking milk from your tatas. The big difference is you don't see your nipple in your baby's mouth while nursing. Watching while you feel your nipple sucked through the clear plastic is strange. You look like you are a cow hooked up at the dairy farm. If you stick with it, you will get used to it and won't even pay attention anymore. It can be uncomfortable, but for me, not nearly as painful as nursing can be. Make sure you use the right size cone. Your nipples get huge during pregnancy and are still that way during nursing. The cones come in different sizes; don't think what came with the pump you are using is your only option. You want there to be enough room for your nipples to fully come through the plastic tube area and not get rubbed raw.

I know some moms who never pumped, just breastfed whenever needed. The problem is that you can never leave your baby for more than a couple of hours. If you want to supplement with formula in a bottle, then issue resolved. You may, however, still need to pump while you are out so you don't come back home looking like you got sprayed down with a garden hose. If you want your baby to just have breast milk, and you plan on leaving him or her with someone for the day or going back to work before you switch to formula, then you are going to need a pump. You need to pump when away from your baby in order to keep your milk supply up. Even if you have tons of breast milk in the fridge or freezer, don't try to go without pumping. Your boobs will start to wean themselves and your milk supply will start to diminish.

I recommend getting a very nice dual pump if you are going to be pumping daily. If you are lucky enough like me to have one or two given to you, then that's great. Just make sure you get all new tubing for it. You can also buy all the other accessories new, too. I got everything for mine from the lactation department at my hospital, but they are available in baby sections at most stores, too. I am currently pumping every three to four hours. I can do it so quick now that it's no hassle at all. I keep everything ready and clean on my bathroom counter. He is also eating every three to four hours, so I am still staying one feeding ahead. This way I can just set it out at room temperature and it's ready whenever he is. Time can get away from you, and I like to be able to go ahead and give him a bottle whenever he's ready. It can be very stressful to have to pump while he is screaming at the top of his lungs ready to eat. If I am leaving him with Ryan or anyone else, I always leave the next bottle ready to feed and several of my milk bags in the fridge. You can buy bags that you can connect directly to your pump, but they never worked well for me; I like the hard plastic bottles that I can hold in place better.

I always take the pump with me, so if I'm not back within four hours I can pump while I am out. Most of the time I plug my pump into an electrical outlet to get power, but they have options for on the go. You don't always have an outlet available, so the nice pumps have that covered. There is a battery pack you can use that takes about forty-eight AA batteries, well maybe not quite that many, but a lot. I use that occasionally, but the batteries run down quickly and I can't afford to buy batteries and diapers weekly at this point. The car charger works best for me. I know, I know, it sounds crazy to pump in your car, but it's no big deal once you're used to it. I'm good at picking very discreet places where no one can see. I work out of my car, so if I was going to continue to give my kid's breast milk, this is what I had to do.

With my first, I would go back to the office when needed, but that is too much trouble. I would take everything in, and then sit in an office behind a closed door pumping away. It is so strange to hear your co-workers going on about their day while you are "milking." Our doors didn't have locks, so I taped to the door a sign that said "Breastfeeding—Do Not Enter." I figured that way people had been warned. I was paranoid someone would forget or the office manager wouldn't mention it to someone who didn't see me go in the office. Nobody ever opened the door, thank goodness! This was just too much trouble, though, so I started pumping on the go.

I had several regular places on my route that I could go. If you have to do this, too, churches work great. Small churches are the best because nobody is around except Sunday mornings and Wednesday nights. They are usually vacant on weekdays. I would keep my little cooler and cold packs in the car, and it didn't take much time at all. I would always have gallon zip-top baggies to put all my milk-splashed cones and containers into. I know this sounds like a lot, but you just get used to packing it up every morning with all the other baby stuff. I did it so much longer with my first because I didn't have two kids to handle in the mornings. It was too much effort with my second, and that's when I just nursed twice a day and supplemented with formula.

I am a huge advocate on not giving up on breast milk if nursing doesn't work for you. Your baby gets the benefit of all the good stuff that's in there, and you save money by not having to buy formula for a while! You also get the benefit of losing baby weight quicker. It just sucked the weight right off me, and I could still eat whatever I wanted. The problem is you can't always eat for two. As soon as you stop nursing, all those extra calories can't escape out your boobs, so they go straight to your thighs!

If you decide to use a pump, you will also have the option of drinking alcohol while breastfeeding. I still call it breastfeeding, even though it is not direct. I have not had an adult beverage or as we call them in front of our kids "a mommy/daddy drink" since I have had this baby. I think it's about time for a margarita night! You can just pump and dump if you have a beverage. I have always heard that if you are feeling the effects of alcohol, then it can be transferred to your baby. I never take the chance of giving my child breast milk if I have consumed alcohol even hours before. I always have a very large stockpile of milk, so it's not that big of a deal. Soon, my husband will no longer have his official DD. He jokes that I have been the designated driver for years now. It seems as though I have either been pregnant or nursing for the last six years straight!

Get ready for leakage! Even if you've got your production and how much the baby needs in synch, there's still a high chance of leakage. Wear some sort of breast pad. I like the disposable kind because all pads smell like sour milk. It's disgusting to keep them around for any amount of time before you wash them, and I feel like the cloth ones don't soak it up as well. Inevitably, you will probably leak on yourself in public. Keep an extra shirt on hand for emergencies. I had a fall baby this time, so that makes it so much nicer. I am wearing layers all the time, so, if I soak through, it's not that big of a deal. I always have a hoodie or a jacket nearby, so I can just put that on to cover my wet pancakes if needed. You know when your milk is going to let down. You feel that warm sensation, so it's time to stop what you are doing and feed or pump before you have boob showers!

My sister had her first baby and was out shopping at a children's clothing store for my nephew. She was new at this, like all us first-time moms. She didn't realize just what happens when you're overdue for a feeding. If you feed your child every three to four hours, then your boobs are ready then, too. Don't think if you've got a mommy's day out and your baby covered with breast milk in the fridge you can wait until you get home. You better be taking your pump out with you! My sister had my nephew with her at the time and he started crying. A baby crying makes your milk start pouring. She started leaking everywhere. So she said she immediately just took all the baby clothes she was going to buy and pressed them up against her, then went to the checkout and paid for all her milk-soaked new baby clothes. Oh well, if it's got to happen, I'm sure a children's clothing store is much more understanding than some other places might be.

When you are trying to nurse, sometimes, you are so ready that as the baby latches on you spray the baby down first. I used to do this to my middle child all the time. She couldn't get on quick enough before my boobs would start a little sprinkler. It is very funny, but it can be very stressful at the time. I shot her in the eye and on the forehead. The milk was coming out so much faster than she could get her little lips in place. So many times I had to give her a quick sponge bath right after I fed her to keep her from souring. When that is happening you need more than just a burp cloth for nursing, you need a towel! If you feel like you are that full before you start, just put a towel on your shoulder for quick clean-up. You may want it for yourself, too. Milk won't only shoot out at the baby, but it will run down your side onto your clothes. I would sometimes even shoot a little in the towel, then try and put her face in place real quick before I got going again to try and prevent the slip and slide. Most recently, when I tried to nurse our baby boy, I was sitting in the living room. My husband was sitting in the chair right beside me. I've got our baby next to my chest, and I was just spraying him down with milk all over his face. No way he was latching on; I just thought maybe I could try this breastfeeding thing one more time. Ryan was saying, "Stop doing that to our son! Your boob is bigger than his head. He can't even get out of the way!" Yeah, that was my last attempt.

If your milk comes in this extreme, your new perfume will be sour milk for several weeks. If you have a great nursing experience like I did with my second, you will eventually even out to where your body isn't producing milk this crazy. I still wore breast pads just in case, but very seldom leaked. When it was time to nurse, she nursed, and my boobs didn't think I had triplets to feed!

I recommend using a waterproof mattress pad on your bed the first couple of weeks. Just in case you bleed through or saturate your nursing pads, you are covered.

Now, don't think it's this way for everyone. I've got a lot of friends whose milk never came in enough to even give breast milk. Some gave up quickly, but others pumped like crazy still with no success. Just go to formula or be one of those weirdos buying other people's breast milk online. If you have done this or are considering it, sorry, but I personally think that's insane. Although I could have probably made lots of extra money if I just pumped a few extra times a day!

I have chosen to stay in a different room from my husband right now. I'm trying to make sure he gets a decent night's sleep because he is the only one working at the moment. And again, I'm trying to preserve our sex life. When you are lying beside someone who reeks of sour milk, it's not very appealing. He doesn't seem to like it when my boobs wet the bed! I just thought I would keep all this fun to myself while the situation is so extreme.

I know some of you will argue that he needs to be a part of every aspect and needs to help in the middle of the night with feedings. Realistically, what can he do when you are nursing? He could be the errand boy and get what I need, but he can't pump or nurse for me. There is no sense in both of us being up several times a night. Trust me, he's seen plenty to know it's not easy during the night, and I know he appreciates all I'm doing at this stage. He knows I could handle it very differently and has thanked me on several occasions for doing it this way. You both don't need to be groggy, frustrated, sleep-deprived parents. It works for me to be in a separate room, but I don't want to be one of "those" ladies who think my way of doing things is the only advice you should take. Just do whatever works for you when it comes to sleeping arrangements!

When you are trying to wean yourself, you have some options to help. You can always try placing cabbage leaves on your boobs. I never did this myself, but I know several people who used this immediately when their milk came in because they knew they were not going to nurse. They say it works; it's just a little strange and I think it would smell awful. The best way for me is to gradually eliminate one feeding at a time until your milk is gone. Just replace one feeding with a bottle; it won't take long and your body will adjust. I always eliminate night feedings first, so I can try and get more sleep. Hopefully, your baby will adjust to this, too! I weaned myself to only two feedings a day when I went back to work with my second. I would just pump or nurse first thing in the morning and before I went to bed. This way my baby still got some breast milk until the milk finally just dried up. Your tatas will be uncomfortable and weird for a little while. You will get your normal boobs back again one day, but definitely not as perky as before baby. They will be recognizable again and not veiny, warm mom boobs that can shoot milk across the room!

My oldest had already been exposed to me pumping. She had seen me do it with her little sister. She asked lots of questions! She always asked if it hurt. I would catch her holding the cups to her chest pretending she was pumping. She would also walk around "feeding" stuffed animals or baby dolls shoved up her shirt. She knew all about it when it was time for her baby brother to nurse, so it wasn't out of the norm at all. I recently asked her if she was going to pump with her babies so she could give them mommy milk, too. She immediately said, "No, that is disgusting!" That was not the response I expected, and I didn't even know she knew the word disgusting.

Little sister had never seen me pump before. Her vocabulary is growing, but she isn't able to communicate like big sister with a baby in the house. I wanted to show her what it was so she didn't freak out the first time she saw me doing it, so I called her into the bathroom. I explained to her what it was and why I was doing it. I showed her all the parts and put it all together. She shook her head yes like she completely understood all I was doing. I attached them to my boobs and turned it on and it didn't phase her one bit. She watched the milk squirt out of my nipples into the container. I told her the milk was for baby brother and she nod her head in agreement. You would have thought she had already seen this a hundred times.

At almost two years old, my little girl loves to dance. She watches her big sister and wants to do all the same moves. She's got rhythm, too. I don't know many other two year olds who can clap while keeping a beat! Whenever she hears any music, she immediately starts jamming out. Now came the pump dance. If you have ever seen or used a pump before, you know they make a funny sound. The strong pumps make a suction sound while you pump, like a beat. It's a pump rhythm like shoo, huh, shoo, huh, shoo, huh, shoo, huh. Well, she starts by bending her knees every time it makes the pump sound. She is bending her knees to the beat, and it is adorable! I will turn up the pump speed and the pump rhythm goes faster, too. She always keeps the beat with bending her knees. She pumps her knees while I pump my tatas to the same rhythm. I have gone into the bathroom where I keep the pump and busted her with the pump turned on doing her pump dance. It is hilarious! It doesn't come quite this natural for mom and dad to see the pump in action. Using a pump is awkward and kind of scary at first. Nobody is quite ready to have to milk their boobs. I wish it was as normal to me the first time as it seemed to be to my two year old when she saw it.

Chapter 8
Hormones

I am writing this when I am actually out of the house running errands. I thought I could get some things recorded during my drive time. Watch out world, here we come! I don't get out very much these days. I love being at home right now and being off work. But, sometimes, being at home just gets to me and I get cabin fever. I need to bust out. Today is one of those days! Usually, all I do is drive to the elementary school and then right back home, but not today. I've got two of the three kids with me right now because my oldest is at kindergarten. The three children and I have not made any public appearances. It might be awhile, I don't think anyone is quite ready. I know I'm not ready yet! I just plan accordingly right now. Like today, I'm out with my almost two year old and newborn. I'm first only running errands where I don't actually have to get out of the car. I know, it's kinda sad to hear. I feel like I've got all this freedom just because I left my house and I'm not even going to get out of the car right now, or if I do, it will be for a few seconds with my kiddos in sight.

Then I'm going to go out to my parents' house. I plan to have lunch with them and leave the two year old there for a long nap. Then my baby and I will pick up the oldest from school and I will actually run errands where we go into places. It's much easier to run errands with just two of the kids, and easiest with the oldest and youngest. My middle is a typical two year old, and it's dangerous just to get through a parking lot at this stage. God love her, but she is my little wild woman right now! Unless she is buckled into something, she is on the run!

I remember talking to my friends about the very first time we left the house by ourselves after having our first child. It's so funny that years after this happens several of my friends still remembered the feeling. Leaving your baby for the first time is hard. Even if you are leaving him or her for a short period of time with your husband, you think the baby needs you constantly. Your husband will take down your list of instructions and act like he's going to do it that way. As soon as you're gone "dad's way" kicks in. It's not any better or worse than what you do, just different. This will drive you crazy at first if you actually figure out what's going on. But you will learn to love it. The fact that your hubby learns what works best for him and the baby is a good thing. It may work better a different way than you do things, and it's great that he has enough time with the baby to figure that out. Don't always correct or try to change what he does; just watch and love that he is figuring out his own way that works best for him.

The first time out alone for one of my friends was a Target trip. Mine was to run errands, too, but I couldn't tell you where I was going. What I do remember, we both had in common. She said as soon as she got in her car she blasted her radio and rolled down the windows. I did the same thing. I remember turning up my radio and jamming out like I hadn't done since I was a teenager. I don't know what it is about rolling your windows down and turning your radio up that gives you such a sense of freedom. It sounds silly, but it's what we both needed. Unless the weather doesn't allow, I highly recommend it for you, too!

I've talked mostly about the physical craziness that goes on with your body right after you have your baby. Now it's time to talk about hormones and your mental status. This is probably the hardest part to overcome. It's a matter of making sense out of having a child and coming home to your life being completely upside down and unlike anything you know. You and your husband/baby's daddy are working together to try and figure out how to take care of this baby. Yes, you are leaking, bleeding, cramping, and on top of all that you have to figure all this out in your head. It would be hard enough mentally to completely prepare for a child without your body going through what it just did to get this baby here. Aside from your body in this state of turmoil, your hormones are also trying to figure out what just happened. They are going from pregnancy to postpartum and you can feel like you are going insane. It's a lot for us all to experience.

For a little while when you first come home, you lose yourself. Get ready for this; it is normal. You will hear about the baby blues and postpartum depression, and it can be a very real thing. If you feel like you are having symptoms where you truly feel depressed and you can't shake yourself out of it, then please ask for help. Go see your doctor and explain what is going on, and get the help you need. If you think of doing anything harmful to yourself or your baby, go seek help. This does happen to some new moms and needs to be addressed immediately. I think this can happen to new dads as well as new moms. When your life as you know it has changed, we all react differently. This change is definitely for the better and everyone will see that in time. For some, it takes longer than others.

I know a friend who did not feel an instant bond with their child. She actually wanted nothing to do with the baby. No desire to hold or nurture her newborn. If you find yourself in this position, do not ignore it. Talk to your husband, your family, your doctor and get the help you need. You will look back on this soon and realize how quickly this time goes. At the moment, it can feel like you are never going to find yourself again. It can be extremely overwhelming and you do not have to suffer through these emotions alone. The fact is that you can no longer live your life the way you know it. Your routine, your social life, your *everything* is different than it was just a few short weeks ago. You can feel like a prisoner in your own home. Again, if you are not able to keep it in perspective and handle it on your own, ask for help!

It's no big deal if you need help. So what if you have to pop an antidepressant or you need to go to counseling for a little while; you will be doing what is best for yourself and your family. It will make this experience better and your family stronger in the long run. Your spouse needs to be included in this, too. His world is also being rocked. He also needs to seek help if needed or be there to support you.

The time where you completely lose yourself is very brief and happens most often with the birth of your first child. There is a good chance you will be able to relate. Like anything, experience is the best teacher. Once you have more children, you know what to expect and you are not anywhere near as overwhelmed. You already know your life is about to become taking care of baby 24/7. The balancing act is easier even though you have two kids at two different stages. I think the older sibling actually helps distract from baby around the clock. When it's your first baby, you may feel like you are never going to be yourself again. Your body has gone whacko. You don't feel attractive. You don't feel feminine. Your day-to-day life is holding, feeding, and changing this newborn, and you can start to function on autopilot. This is the time to bond. This is the time to cherish every moment. As much as I try to prepare you and as much as you logically know this, it probably won't happen. Your emotions won't let it.

You will wish this time away like so many of us moms already have. You will have lack of sleep and be so ready to move onto sleeping all night and the next baby stage. Just wait until you do have more children, you will get it all so much better then. You will learn that you have to appreciate this newborn time before it is gone. I so wish I didn't wish all this away with my first child. I just wanted to get back to feeling like me again and went through the motions until I started to get there. With my two other children, I loved every second. Right now, I cherish every time I get to hold this sweet baby. Don't get me wrong. I could do without holding him quite so many times during the night, but I am not wishing it away!

Every time I look into those sweet little eyes and capture the stage he is in right now is irreplaceable. He is going to grow up right before me even quicker than his older sisters. I know this is my last one, and I don't want to miss a thing! He will be a toddler in a blink. It happens so fast. You hear people say that, but when they are newborn sometimes the days and nights seem never ending. You just don't truly get it! Once you are through it, you can't get it back. Each and every stage that you think is so hard is also jam packed with precious memories and milestones. Take lots of pictures. Take lots of videos. Look at that sweet little face and soak up as much as you can.

It's a lot easier to say that now, when I have already experienced it. In the midst of it, there's no better way to describe it than feeling like you have lost yourself. And, in reality, you have lost your prior self. The life you have lived up to this point is gone. It will never be the same. It just takes a little while to realize it's a wonderful thing. Like any major change, it's not always easy, even though it is for the better. I think some of the baby blues is mourning that you have completely closed the former chapter of your life. You can no longer be independent, going where you want when you want without considering another little one constantly. The rest of your life, your focus, and priorities will be different. When it happens literally overnight, it's a lot to take in at one time. But what you will gain from motherhood will make you so much better than you have ever been before!

We waited a little while to start our family. Ryan and I started dating in high school. We dated for eight years until we got married in 2003. We went on lots of trips and spent many years together with it being just the two of us. We had our first child in 2006, only three years after we had been married, but more than ten years after we met. I think it's important to have time to really get to know your spouse before starting a family. Depending on how old you are when you meet and get married, it might not be practical. We all have biological clocks ticking, but I'm glad we had this time together. I think the younger you are, the harder it may be to move to this stage. We had our crazy times. We were ready to settle down and give up the night life. I was twenty-nine when I had my first child. If I would have had a baby in my early twenties, it would have been very hard to close that chapter of my life. Just know, whatever your stage or whatever age you are, it is worth it! You will get a social life back, but your idea of having a fun night will turn into watching your baby "army crawl" around your living room. This is a good thing. God has placed this baby with you at this time in your life, and you will be a much better person because of that.

There is nothing better than being a parent. You will not truly understand this until you have your baby. I don't care how many close family and friends you have with babies. Until you experience becoming a mom and dad for yourself, you will not understand it. I thought I knew what love was. I am so in love with my husband. I love my mom, dad, sister and her family. I married into an amazing family that I love. I have three nieces and two nephews who I love like crazy. But it's a different kind of love that you feel for your own child. I think it's one of the only times that you can begin to know God's love. That is the best way to describe a love that a mother and father feel for their own child. It is awesome to experience it!

Initially, however, you may not be there. Some people can look at their own child and immediately feel that bond and that love. That's how it's supposed to work, right? It would be great if it worked that way for everyone, but sadly, it doesn't. It can take a while until you are at this point with your baby. Sometimes, the connection just takes a little longer. Either way, whatever you experience, it's okay and it is normal. You will get there with your child. If at first you are more concentrated on how to take care of this baby and the bonding hasn't set in yet, it will. I know some moms are intimidated about caring for the baby and can't embrace it fully. If this happens to you, there is a good chance when you have another child it will come much quicker. Don't worry, you will connect. Your body is reeling from childbirth and your hormones are fluctuating off the charts. You are given this newborn child who you are supposed to take care of, and sometimes what should be a time of bliss can be filled with fear and anxiety. Talk this time through with friends and family and get as much support as you need.

Your hormones will be out of control for a little while. During pregnancy, you have already experienced this. I'm going to call it pregnancy personality because while you are pregnant it is not always a true representation of what your personality normally is. At least for me it's not. With my first two, my pregnancies were very easy. Not many symptoms, very little nausea. I felt good through most of it. Low energy was my biggest problem. I was, however, overly emotional. Both of them were girls and I don't know if this had to do with extra amounts of estrogen in my system. But with both of them, I would cry so easy. Things that would never even phase me before would make me sob! I was a mess listening to certain songs or watching shows and movies. I'm sure many of you can relate; this is what we are always told to expect with our pregnancy emotions.

With my third child, I did not have the same experience. Not sure if it's because he was a boy or just the fact that I was stressed having two other children while going through a pregnancy, but it was very different. I wasn't emotional. I liked to call it hormonal, but in reality it was bitchy! I was so bitchy! And I wonder if it really does have to do with having boys versus girls. Maybe all that testosterone wasn't getting along with me and turned me into a bitch. I asked my sister and several friends who have had both sexes, and they didn't notice that big of a difference. I'm telling you, I would speak my mind about anything at any time. This is not like me! I will try to be as polite as possible in any situation. I will look at something bad and try my best to turn or present it in a positive light. At work I would do my very best to let things go. I am usually a laid back person and have the mentality that life is way too short to get worked up over little things. I couldn't find that perspective these last few months.

There are very few people who genuinely get on my nerves, but everybody did during this pregnancy! Nobody could say or do the right thing. I knew that it was me, not them, but they still annoyed the hell out of me! I just bit my tongue. My poor husband got it all when I was at home. I wouldn't hold anything back with him. Sorry Ryan, I know you got the brunt of everyone who annoyed me for a few months. He could tell you that there was quite a difference in how I acted this last pregnancy. Toward the end of the pregnancy, I didn't feel so angry all the time. I thought I had finally gotten back to myself. I think I probably had just gotten used to being a bitch, so it didn't phase me anymore. I could have asked Ryan, but I'm sure whatever he would have said would have ticked me off at the time!

After you have the baby, who knows what your emotions will do. You may snap at everybody about everything. You may be a sweet emotional new mom crying happy tears all the time. Your baby's daddy just has to hang in there with you! By that point, he will have had the pregnancy personality warning. He will be used to you being somewhat of an emotional mess. It takes some time for our hormones to work themselves out. Just know everyone is overwhelmed. You are not alone. You will get through it! It is worth every single hormonal second! You will realize this, too, and your crazy hormones will float into this same fog with all your body troubles. Don't lose sight of this ultimate gift you have been given, and I promise you will find yourself again. In a short time, you may hear someone else talk about how rough it is mentally when you bring a baby home. You won't even be able to relate anymore. You will be so removed and enjoying your baby at whatever stage he or she has begun.

I have debated whether or not to include this in the book. I skimmed over it earlier in this chapter, but I've decided it needs attention. With Ryan's permission, here we go. . . .

I mentioned that both mom and dad may suffer from some sort of postpartum depression or baby blues, and we experienced it firsthand. The birth of our second child took its toll on my husband. I was so much more prepared and everything was easier for me. I didn't hurt as bad, nursing came naturally, and the baby slept better. I was prepared for at least the same amount of stress and pain as the first, and was pleasantly surprised at how much easier everything was that time. I could truly enjoy those first few weeks with our newborn and soak it up. It had the opposite effect on Ryan.

He is a wonderful dad and went straight into daddy mode with our first. We were on opposite shifts, so even at three months, he kept her all day while I was at work. He had no anxiety about doing this and bonded so well with her even when she was only a few months old. I've learned that it usually takes men much longer to bond than women. We are more likely to look into those newborn eyes and connect. Dads love their newborn babies, but they usually need some sort of response from them. Once they start to giggle and play, dads have a much easier time bonding. Up to this point, they usually just see the baby as an eating, pooping, burping machine and can't bond yet.

Ryan lost himself after our second baby was born. At first, he reacted very similarly to when our first was born. He was all about helping and spending time with her and her older sister. Then something changed. He loved his family including this new baby girl, but he didn't want anything to do with us. It was like he completely rebelled from fatherhood. This didn't happen until she was a couple months old. I had never heard of this before, so I started researching postpartum in males and it is a very real thing. Their lives have also been turned upside down, and all the attention is on baby and mom. I don't know if they are ever even asked how it is affecting them. Ryan just shut down. He wouldn't involve himself with our family and even started staying away as much as possible. He would work overtime, go to friends' houses on the way home, stay out late with the guys. Anything possible to stay away from the house. I think the fact that this was our second child had a lot to do with it.

The only thing I could get out of him was that he couldn't handle being with both of them alone. I would leave for small amounts of time and come home, and he would look like a zombie staring into space. Kids were fed, diapers changed, but he did not enjoy one moment of it. He couldn't handle two kids at two different stages. Like most men, Ryan is project driven. Give him a task and he doesn't want to stop until he finishes it. He is focused and determined. I am the scatter brained multitasker. I guess we fit into our assumed gender roles. It doesn't bother me at all to start laundry, then have to help a kid go poop, feed a crying baby, then back to laundry again. It drives him insane!

I think because he didn't enjoy being with the kids anymore, he wanted his former independent life back. I don't know how many times he voiced this frustration to me; he knew he should be acting differently, but couldn't help it. I would try my best to talk things through with him, but he didn't want to hear it. What did I do? I prayed. Prayed more than I ever have prayed. For my husband, for my family, but most of all for our marriage. I didn't care how he acted or how long he acted like it; I was never giving up on us. I didn't tell many people about this. My sister is the one who helped me get through this, and I will never know how to truly thank her. I don't know what I would have done without her. This lasted for months. I tried to get him to go to the doctor or counseling, but he refused. I didn't want to push him away more, so I let that go for the moment and just kept praying.

Then as quick as it set in, it was gone. Overnight, I had my Ryan back! I know it was baby blues! It was a mental disconnect that was his response to a new family dynamic that he couldn't handle. With our third, no issues at all. It's already so much clearer that his comfort level is where it should be. He is a very hands-on dad and is enjoying every minute, well almost every minute, of family life. You may think his bond may somehow be different with our second because of what he experienced. That is not the case! She is daddy's girl, and he wouldn't have it any other way!

I don't know just how common it is for men to go through this. Like most things, once you start talking about it, you find out you are one of many who has gone through something similar. I didn't share this with many people out of respect for my husband. Now on the other side, we both feel like we need to talk about it. In case you also experience this, we want you to know you are not alone. Try not to get frustrated with your husband/baby's daddy, just help him through this time. Think about what you would need from him if you were going through this experience. It doesn't matter if it's the mom or dad, parenthood is life changing and can have major effects on all of us. Just love him more than you ever have and seek help if needed.

Chapter 9

NICU

I only experienced the NICU with my third child. The NICU is the abbreviation for neonatal intensive care unit. It is so hard to have a child there! I had only actually been in a NICU one other time and always had compassion for those parents with little ones there. I became one of "those" parents, and it absolutely sucked! Like everything else that doesn't go exactly as planned, you never think it will happen to you. Then when it does, you have more understanding and love for all those babies than you ever thought imaginable. So many are so fragile and so tiny and I knew I couldn't, but I wanted to know the diagnosis and story of each and every one of those sweet little babies. I found myself asking the nurses questions about other babies, and of course they would remind me that they couldn't share any details.

I couldn't believe my sweet little boy was lying in the intensive care unit with oxygen, IVs, and a feeding tube. Everything about it is hard! Our little boy had very minimal problems in comparison to the other babies, but as long as he was there, I was extremely worried! At one point they had found an "air pocket" in his lung. He was already there because he had too much fluid in his lungs, or as they referred to it they were "cloudy." The last update I had gotten he was going in the right direction, and then they started talking about this new pocket they had found. I remember asking if this was something he might not overcome. I am tearing up right now just thinking about that moment. I had no idea how serious it might be. When things go wrong when your baby is already in the NICU, it is scary! They assured me it was only a minor setback, and he would just have to stay a little longer to recover.

Up to that point, I knew he was there for a very common problem, and although I was worried sick, I never had the thought that he may not survive. That's the first thing that came into my head the moment they mentioned something additional was wrong. I quickly learned that it was not life threatening and all he needed was time. I can't explain how emotionally draining the days in the NICU were for me, and I had it easy in comparison to those other parents. Our baby boy looked like a giant in the NICU. Most of those babies were preemies and weighed only a couple pounds. He was born weighing 7 pounds, 5 ounces. He would have looked very average in the regular nursery, but in the NICU he was huge! I almost felt bad that I was going into visit my baby, who looked so much healthier than most of the other sweet babies there. I don't know what the average length of stay is in a NICU, but I know some of those babies have to be there for months. Eight days was too long for me!

Our baby was born at thirty-eight weeks. This is supposed to be full term, but our baby boy wasn't ready. My doctors decided to induce because of his kidney hydronephrosis (kidney blockage is the easiest way to explain it) and prevention of another gigantic 11-pound baby like his big sister. The high-risk obstetrician was very worried about his kidney and wanted an ultrasound done immediately after his birth. These images were supposed to be sent to the pediatric urology specialist while he was still in the hospital to determine if he would need surgery right away. This baby was not ready to be born! He needed a couple more weeks with me to get ready for his big arrival. We had forced him to start the delivery process, and he was not planning on making an exit this early. After a full day of labor, I wouldn't even dilate more than five centimeters and his heart rate was dropping, so it was C-section time. I'm sure it's a combination of his lungs not being ready and fluid not getting pushed out like it should during a vaginal delivery that produced fluid in his lungs. It can be known as "wet" or "cloudy" lungs, but this is what landed him in the NICU. Images were taken the day after birth of his kidney troubles, but that was all secondary to his current lung situation. I was worried that he might need emergency medical attention right after birth, but I never dreamed it would be for anything other than his kidney.

He could not keep a good oxygen level. I got to hold him the first time I went to the NICU to see him and had no idea how closely the nurses were watching his vital signs. He couldn't take any exertion at all without his oxygen levels dropping quickly. I wasn't able to hold him again for days. They wouldn't even take him out of the bassinet. They had to put a feeding tube in because even taking a bottle was too much exertion. The IV placement was the hardest for me. He wouldn't stop messing with it and trying to pull it out, so they had to keep moving it. They warned me before they had to put it on his head to keep it in. At least he was no longer messing with it all the time. You are not supposed to see your newborn baby attached to all these machines with all these tubes. All I could do was watch him and occasionally take his temperature or change his diaper. I just wanted to be doing something for him. He needed to be held, but if that wasn't possible I wanted any chance I could get to have contact with him. I would stand over him and rub his little leg wanting so badly to pick him up.

I pumped every three hours around the clock, and my milk was in big time. They said it would take five days with a C-section, but I had milk flowing after just two days. This was something I could provide for my baby, so I was pumping like clockwork. I would label the breast milk and bring it to the NICU each time. They would put it in their refrigerator so they could give it to him. The nurses would laugh at me every time I showed up with my milk to drop off. They couldn't believe how much I was able to pump. It was the one thing I could actually do for my child. When we left they gave me the ridiculous amount of milk they had not used. I had my husband bring a little six-pack cooler thinking that would hold it. After a full week of me pumping around the clock, we needed the biggest cooler we own. I have a wonderful freezer supply for whenever I am away from our baby or want to have a few drinks.

I was elated the day we got the news it was time to plan for discharge! I was in for one of my many daily visits, and the doctor was giving me my report and asked, "Are you ready to take him home?" I had no idea whether he was going to be there for two or ten more days, and I know I squealed! Again, I felt horrible for those other moms. I almost think she should have told me privately, but I know that's just not how they give reports. The NICU is very similar to most hospital nurseries, just a lot more high-tech equipment and those babies stay around the clock. It's one big open room with bassinets or incubators lining the walls. There were several moms around visiting their babies when I got my news. After I stopped celebrating, I saw them looking at me. They knew it would be a long time before they got the same news. So many of those tiny preemies would have to be there for many more weeks, if not months. I thought to myself how hard it must be for them. They see other babies come in, stay for however many days, then go home. In the meantime, they are still making daily visits to their babies, while they try to function in some sort of normalcy. So much time has passed that some of those moms are back to work and somewhat of a normal routine while their sweet babies are still stuck in the hospital. It's not fair, but they know the baby is where he or she needs to be at that time.

There is a fairly common term used in the NICU. I had never heard it before this experience, but when this happened we heard it multiple times. We even heard it from friends who had some sort of NICU background or had similar situations with their own child. The term is *wimpy white male*. I've been told and read about the fact that white male babies are more prone to needing help if born early. For some reason, who knows why, their lungs are not always fully developed. There is a much higher chance that a premature or preterm white boy will need oxygen more than girls or other races. I understand that it's very common to see these little boys in the NICU with oxygen. I was not ready to hear that term while our baby was struggling. My husband wanted to take out the nurse who first used that term in front of him.

This was our precious baby boy. He was not healthy and had to go straight to intensive care. He was fighting to be able to breathe on his own. He was our brave and courageous son hooked up to all these tubes. We were very nervous about him having to go to the NICU and were praying for his strength. And here comes a nurse joking about him being another "wimpy white male" when we were in visiting. I know that they use that term among themselves all the time, and I know that our baby fit the description very well; however, the nurses do not need to say this in front of the baby's parents. If I would have heard the term before it was used to describe our son, it probably wouldn't have bothered me so bad. My husband still comes unglued if you mention it. He did not appreciate anyone calling our newborn son "wimpy" at the time. Just a warning in case you find yourself in the same situation!

Everything is so different if your baby has to go to the NICU. They knew as soon as they got our boy in the nursery and started checking his vitals that he needed help. They put him in my arms after the C-section, and that was it. I never even got to hold him in the recovery room. Ryan was in the well baby nursery with him with all our family watching through the windows when he could not maintain a healthy oxygen level. They immediately took him to the NICU. The next time I saw our baby is when I was doing well enough to go to the NICU with Ryan to visit him. The NICU is monitored very closely and has very limited visitation. I know that this is necessary for the well-being of these sweet new lives, but it is like having your baby in Fort Knox in comparison to your own hospital room.

At our hospital, very few people are allowed in at all and only two at one time. You are allowed to visit and stay with your baby outside of two-hour windows while shift change is happening. You have to stop and wash your hands and arms up to your elbows in the sinks provided before you walk in. I am very glad that they are so protective of visitors, but it is the constant reminder of how different your baby is from the others. I was blessed to have two other babies who were very healthy and were able to come right back into my arms after their first nursery visit. Even so, I resented the moms who had their babies with them in their rooms.

Only grandparents, aunts, and uncles were included on "our list" for the NICU. No one else who came to see me in the hospital got to see my handsome little man. What really sucked is neither did his big sisters! No children were allowed in the NICU at this time due to flu season. They never got to even meet their little brother until he came home more than a week after he was born. My husband went back to work, my oldest was going to school every day, and our baby wasn't home yet.

Our five year old just happened to have a school family tree project that same week. She brought home a construction paper leaf that she was supposed to put pictures of her family on and take back to school. At this point, I had been discharged and was coming home in the evenings to spend time with the girls and sleep before going back to the hospital the next morning. I got one of the pictures printed of our baby boy and big sister included the baby brother she had not yet met on the leaf. She was so proud, and I was so angry that she hadn't even gotten to see him for herself yet. It is the sweetest picture of him with his little oxygen tube up his nose.

I took several pictures of him while he was in the NICU. He had oxygen and IVs most of the time and for several days a feeding tube. I knew I needed a picture for the big sister school project, and that day he just had oxygen. I asked the nurses if they could take it off just for a quick picture. They put me in my place very nicely and explained that this is what he looked like at this age and that was not a possibility. I'm embarrassed to even say that I asked that. What was I thinking? My kid looks too sick with oxygen on for his pic. Is it okay if we take it off and let his oxygen level drop a little so he can look cute for the picture? I'm such an idiot! Here's one of many times where I felt like the worst mom ever. Trust me, if you are like the rest of us, you will have several worst-mom-ever moments. They pass quickly and hopefully you have many more kickass-mom moments to compensate!

I brought in several items for our baby to have in the NICU. I wanted something from home surrounding him. My favorite was a canvas that I had gotten for his nursery with the saying "You are a Child of God. You are wonderfully made, dearly loved, and precious in His sight. Before God made you, He knew you . . . there is no one else like you!" I also loved displaying coloring pages that his oldest sister had made just for him. Even though he was there such a short period of time, I wanted him surrounded by things from his home and family. He didn't know the difference, but I did. It made it a little easier to leave him when I had to go.

While I was still in the hospital myself, I was in the NICU with my baby about as often as possible. Then the dreaded day came when I had to leave without him. The experience was heart wrenching! That's the only way I can describe it. If you don't have other children, I'm sure it's even harder. I knew I needed to see my girls and spend some time with them at home. I had already been away from them for five days during my hospital stay, but I didn't want to leave. Actually going in to see him for the last time before they sent me home was so hard! I can't even talk about it. If I didn't have my girls waiting for me at home, I probably would have slept right there in the labor and delivery waiting area. I'm sure my sweet husband would have made me go home and I would have appreciated it at some point, but you do not ever want to leave that hospital without your baby!

At this time, Ryan was back at work and I couldn't drive yet. My in-laws to the rescue! I could not have made everything work without them. If you are dealing with a child in the NICU, this is when you can take up everyone on their offers to help! You want to be at the hospital and you can't drive yourself there. If you've got older kids, you need help with childcare or getting them where they need to be. Hubby is probably back at work, so you need to reach out to your extended family and friends. My in-laws were there to help Ryan and I make it happen every day, and I am so appreciative! My middle child was too little to get in her car seat by herself. So, even if I was going to break all the rules and drive too early, I didn't need to be picking her up yet only days after my C-section. Between my husband and his parents they had it all covered.

You do need to get away from the hospital. You need to sleep in your own bed and spend time at home. Your baby is in good hands, and you can't be right there with him or her all the time, anyway. I would go every morning once big sisters were in place and spend the day hanging out at the hospital. My sister was in town several days during the NICU stay. She or my mom would come over and sit with me, then visit my sweet boy, and we would go to lunch. It's very strange to sit down over lunch at a restaurant across the street while your child is in intensive care. It was all very surreal, but I needed out of the hospital environment periodically.

Remember how I told you I swelled up like a whale after my C-section? Well, I'm sure everyone has the best of intentions, but they need to keep their mouth shut. I was spending one of my campout days in the waiting room in labor and delivery. I was working on baby gift thank-you cards when a random lady asked me when I was going to have my baby. "Look lady, I know I'm as big as a house, but I'm not pregnant anymore. I had my sweet baby, and he's under lock and key, and it's not time for me to see him at the moment. I have to sit out here and wait for you to say something like this to make my hormonal, highly emotional self feel that much better about myself and my situation right now!" That's what went through my head. I, of course, explained very nicely that I had my baby the week before and was there to visit him in the NICU. I then went back to what I was working on hoping nobody else would *ever* ask me any questions because no way did I want to explain myself again. So, if anybody thinks you are still pregnant after you give birth, they don't mean to be rude. You think it is a joyous time for all new moms or moms-to-be in the labor and delivery department, but sadly, that is not always the case.

I was discharged home on a Sunday. I was home for only three nights without my baby, but it was still way too long. Our hospital offers for you to "room in" with your baby once he or she can leave the NICU. I'm not real sure just how common this is in hospitals, but it is a wonderful idea. You and your husband get to go to the hospital and stay overnight with your new baby the night before you bring the baby home. It's a room in the hospital that is set up more like a basic hotel room than a hospital room. You get to stay there with your baby all night long. It helps you get over the nervousness of caring for your baby who has just recovered from complications. He seemed so fragile to me. Even though he was my third child, I was nervous about taking care of him. He had highly trained pediatric nurses watching over him 24/7 since birth and now it was me and my husband's responsibility to make sure he was healthy.

Not only does "rooming in" help with your comfort level, but it gives you an opportunity to bond with your child. Even though our baby was eight days old, we hardly even had the chance to hold him up to this point. We had never had him in the room with us and had only seen him in the NICU. I had no idea this was even available, but I am so grateful it is offered. We were very pleased with the NICU at our hospital. We would have preferred to not ever know about the NICU experience. Since we had to be there, I'm glad it all worked out like it did. Our baby was surrounded by caring, compassionate nurses, who loved on him when we couldn't. Thank you for taking such good care of our baby boy!

Chapter 10
Sex after Childbirth

It's time to talk about sex after childbirth. It is very scary for a new mom! You will not be ready to have sex again the first time you attempt, unless you make your spouse wait a very long time. You are not alone. This is scary for most women. I have talked to my friends about this so much. We were all terrified! After your girl parts have gone through so much trauma, the thought of having sex is revolting. Sorry guys, but it is not appealing in the least. The thought of enjoying sex seems totally foreign. You can't imagine that you will ever actually like having sex again. Right after having a baby you don't feel feminine, and you don't feel pretty. You sure don't want your husband touching you anywhere that is leaking or hurts. It takes some time to get to where you are ready to even attempt sex. I'm not there yet. I couldn't care less right now.

My hubby is going to have to wait awhile, and I didn't even have a vaginal delivery this time. I'm not as weirded out about the actual idea of intercourse because, thankfully, this time my girl parts weren't stretched beyond oblivion. I just have no desire, and it sounds gross right now. My boobs leak all the time, and I've got this extra mushy area on my lower abdomen. It's just not going to happen. My husband and I haven't talked about it yet, but with what I just described, I don't think he's going to be too disappointed.

It's more about just getting your sexuality back with a C-section. Your spouse does need to be understanding about this. He has to be very patient with you. You will get there, but it's not going to happen overnight. I'm so glad I don't have to worry about being freaked out about it hurting this time. You need to wait until your doctor gives you the okay. Do not attempt anything before that point. With a vaginal delivery, it is the absolute last thing on earth you want to do. I've given you all the details on what you go through after you deliver. I would have preferred to wait six months instead of six weeks.

I'm going to share with you the same advice my friends and I have given one another about the first time. *Booze and lube ladies!* You need something to help your anxiety that first time. For me and my friends, alcohol did the trick. Just drink a couple glasses of wine or have a couple beers, whatever is your favorite. You need something to help put you at ease. Just relax and loosen up a little bit! The second piece of advice is lubrication. Whether or not you use lube regularly, use it this time! This definitely helps make it less uncomfortable. This also helps your fear that it is going to hurt. I thought the first time after my oldest was born was going to be awful! I was so nervous and so scared. I boozed and lubed just like my friends told me, and surprisingly, it wasn't that bad! Maybe I was too drunk to remember—just kidding! It's so much worse in our minds than actuality. Although, it will take time until you feel ready to initiate and you are back to a normal sex life. I would wear a bra for months because I was worried about shooting my husband in the face with milk.

Everybody dreads this topic. We don't want that six-week follow-up appointment with the doctor to ever come. Our guys are so excited about this appointment. They know it's time for us to be cleared. Game on! We, on the other hand, are terrified. We are hoping the doctor just might have some reason why we need to hold off for a while. It's a completely different reaction between men and women. Just booze and lube, and it will be just fine.

If you have been with your man for a long time, you may need to remind him about a few things. Sometimes, when you have been married for years, guys forget what it means to have foreplay, especially if you already have children. You have quickies when you get a chance. Most of the time when it is finally just the two of you, you are too tired to do anything but sleep. You need to remind him that you need these extra touches and kisses to get you aroused and get your sexuality back. Your man needs to woo you again. Men sometimes quit wooing. You need to feel loved; you need to feel sexy. Just explain to him that you need all the extras. The little touches and flirting will help encourage your sex life. It won't be long and you will be ready for a quickie too, but hopefully some of the extras will stick long term.

Don't forget about birth control! Your doctor will discuss options at your six-week appointment. Once you have had a successful pregnancy, no matter how hard it was to get pregnant, it can happen again. I know too many people who tried for years to get pregnant and then wound up pregnant shortly after giving birth to their first. Once your body goes through the miracle of childbirth, it knows exactly what to do. Pregnancy can happen so much easier from that point forward. Even if you had an extremely hard time getting pregnant the first time, be ready or take birth control!

I never had a very difficult time getting pregnant, but I did experience miscarriage. I had a miscarriage with my very first pregnancy. It was actually called a blighted ovum. I think I had the same emotional loss that any mom feels with a miscarriage. You test positive on a pregnancy test. Your body has all the symptoms that you have when you are pregnant. Your boobs are sore and start to change appearance quickly. Your uterus is growing, and your clothes are getting tight. You think your pregnancy is well under way. I was eleven weeks along when I found out that my pregnancy had failed. The sperm did fertilize the egg and cells started multiplying. Then it just fizzled out. An actual fetus was never even created. The fertilized egg just stopped developing even before it became an embryo.

We didn't try again for a year. We had a trip planned to Las Vegas, and I knew I was going to be ovulating, so this was the first time we tried again. Our oldest is our Vegas baby. What happens in Vegas did not stay in Vegas for us! We have our sweet baby girl from that trip. With our next baby, we tried for almost six months. I was keeping up with when I should be ovulating, and during that time we had sex every other day like they tell you to do. I always knew just when I was ovulating, but I wasn't paying any attention to forty weeks ahead. That's how we ended up with a December 25 due date. I wouldn't have had it any other way. We got our sweet Christmas baby and brought her home on Christmas Eve.

Our third was a surprise. We were not trying. I thought we were doing pretty good at avoiding the days of ovulation. Then I got lazy about keeping my eye on the calendar. Just in case, we were also using what I like to call the "banking method." What I mean by this is the early withdrawal tactic. I guess we didn't take our money out early enough. We were not using any other form of birth control. I didn't want to get back on the pill and we hate using condoms!

I'm also paranoid about buying condoms. I don't know what it is about buying them. I am a married woman in my mid-thirties, and I still feel so slutty buying condoms. It's not like I'm buying them to use for one-night stands. I just can't handle going through the checkout with them. I immediately feel like a sixteen-year-old girl doing something I am not supposed to do. Why is this? I can go to pick up my birth control pills and it's no big deal. I can have a conversation with the pharmacist about my pills and joke about having more kids. But when I'm in line to buy condoms, I want to be in disguise. I feel like everyone is judging me and making assumptions about what is in my cart. My husband and I used to always joke about what else to buy at the same time just to mess with people. I would never do this, but it is funny. I won't tell you all the things that were on the list, but I'm sure you can come up with your own. I dare you to go buy it all at the same time and see the reaction as you check out. Especially if you are really pregnant right now, I'd give you bonus points for that; it would be hilarious!

Anyway, my husband doesn't like to wear condoms. *Shocker!* I'm sure most men don't. We always had said two maybe three kids. Right after I had my second, I knew I wasn't done. Once Ryan got adjusted to life with two kids, he felt the same way. We would have never planned to have them this close together, but it's exactly what our family needed. We were planning to go on a cruise for our friends' wedding. First trip without the girls and I was worried and excited to be away for that long. I did not want to be on my period while I was on the cruise, and should have already started that month. I don't keep up with my periods exactly unless I am trying to get pregnant. The cruise was getting closer and I still hadn't started. I knew it was time, and I didn't expect to be on my period while we were cruising. I started to wonder if maybe I was pregnant.

I talked to Ryan and had him pick up a pregnancy test. I was so nervous when I peed on that stick, but then, the results were negative. I stared at that pregnancy test and was shocked that I was disappointed. I just knew that I would be relieved, but when the results came back, I wasn't relieved at all. I knew that I was ready to have another baby. Good thing, because a couple days later when I still hadn't started, I took another one. This time, it showed positive results. We were having another baby! I'm so glad that I knew so I didn't drink like a fish on that ship. No regrets, we got our sweet baby boy!

Each of our children are such miracles. God knew what was supposed to happen even though we didn't. What three amazing blessings we have been given! Now it's time for drastic measures. We always said two maybe three kids, never three, maybe four! Our family is complete! My sweet husband is willing to get a vasectomy. My feeling on it is the woman goes through so much with pregnancy and childbirth that it makes sense for the man to step up when it comes to a simple procedure. There are so many options for women, but our surgery requires a much harder recovery, and all the other new gadgets out there to insert make me nervous. I don't want something in me all the time that God didn't put there.

My husband wasn't always willing to have a vasectomy. Initially, he was afraid his junk wouldn't work anymore, and he was way too nervous about having it done. Now, enough family and friends have been through it that he is willing. Our plan is for him to have it within the year. Our baby is only a month old, and we aren't ready for any additional procedures or medical bills at the moment. I plan on getting back on the birth control pill at my six-week appointment and staying on them until we have confirmation that his procedure worked. We are not taking any chances this time!

Once you get beyond your after pregnancy experience, make sure you and your man give each other attention. Being parents makes you closer but also pulls you apart all at the same time. You now share this amazing bond. You have been given a child who is the perfect mix of the two of you. There are so many sweet, funny, and emotional moments you will share watching your baby grow. However, you don't have as much time to do the things the two of you enjoy doing together. Always make time for each other. Don't just be parents and forget to be lovers. Pay the crazy amount of money it takes to have date night from time to time. Go on an overnight getaway with just the two of you on your anniversary or for no special occasion at all. Stay up after the kids go to bed to have some time alone. Make time to keep your marriage strong and passionate. Don't use all your energy on your kids and not have any left for each other. Stay emotionally connected to your husband and make sex a priority!

Conclusion

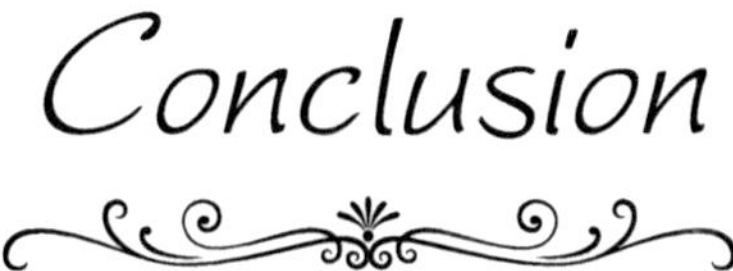

It's now October and I just completed this book. My youngest celebrated his second birthday last Saturday. It's so funny to have listened to myself talking about the time in my life after delivery. I am so far separated from that time, even now. I know I explained in my introduction how I was already experiencing the "memory fog" and couldn't give everything in such detail. I am now even more grateful I captured these moments after listening to all my recordings.

Life is good. Our house is loud, crazy, and at times very stressful, but I can't imagine anything else I'd rather be doing than raising these three kiddos. We stay very busy with a seven, three, and two year old. It is chaos lots of times, but I've learned to embrace the chaos instead of fighting it. I love watching their little personalities and their interaction with one another.

My husband did have his vasectomy so we know our family is complete. It's kind of weird. We know we don't want any more kids. I don't ever even have the thought of wanting another baby, but it's still hard to close that chapter. Just to think I am past the baby-making years is difficult to swallow. We are so blessed, and I know that this is where we are supposed to be at this time in our life. I just still feel like I should be in my twenties, not thirty-six years old!

I was true to my recordings. I did what I said I would do and didn't represent myself any different from what I was experiencing at that moment. Just in case you are wondering, I have felt very secure with myself both physically and emotionally for some time now. I have felt like myself in reference to everything that was discussed in this book for more than a year. I would like to tone and tighten my body in several places, but I have no major body issues. No way am I wearing a bikini, but I'm comfortable with my body. I have no hang-ups with what is left after the C-section. I have a very small scar that is not even very visible. The skin directly above my incision site does not have the full nerve sensation, but it's nothing that bothers me or is even weird.

The "jellyfish" that I referred to in the book hasn't lived on my abdomen since a couple months after my baby boy was born. There is a little extra flap that hangs over where my incision was. It's like when you have on pants that are too tight and your belly folds over the waistline a little bit. (If you can't relate, then you are probably working out so much this will never be an issue for you.) It's just not completely flat in my lower bikini area anymore, but it doesn't bother me one bit. I have not done any major exercise to try and work on it, and I don't know if it can ever tone. I could care less! My hubby is the only one who will ever see it anyway. No, I don't have the body that I used to have, but I have three wonderful kids I would take over a bikini body any day!

One of the things that occurred to me after reading the book was that I focused quite a bit on keeping things from your husband. I don't want you to misunderstand what I mean about this. I mean don't show him everything. There is a difference between sharing and showing. I don't want anyone to fake it and act like everything is okay when it's not. You don't need to pretend you don't hurt or act like you are keeping it together when you are not. I want you to communicate everything to your hubby about what you are going through physically and emotionally, just don't show him all your troubles. You may want to completely keep the bathroom issues from him like I did, but use him for as much support as needed with all you are going through. Every man is different about this, too. Some men aren't phased at all when it comes to all the physical issues. You know your husband; you will do what's right for the two of you!

My recordings make it sound like it was such a difficult time. I have now turned into a mom of little ones who is telling others how quick the crazy times are after just giving birth. I feel like my book makes it sound like my recovery was extreme, but I think I probably handled it like most other new moms, without too many major issues. It's so funny what your perspective is when you are experiencing it. That's why I am so glad I captured this time!

I hope this book has given you some insight into what happens right after delivery. I have loved writing this book and enjoyed listening to myself going through such a special time in my life. Soon you will be looking back with a different perspective too and telling everyone, "It's not that bad." It's comical how this time now seems like a blink in time, and I was able to write an entire book on the subject. Thank you for letting me share my story with you.

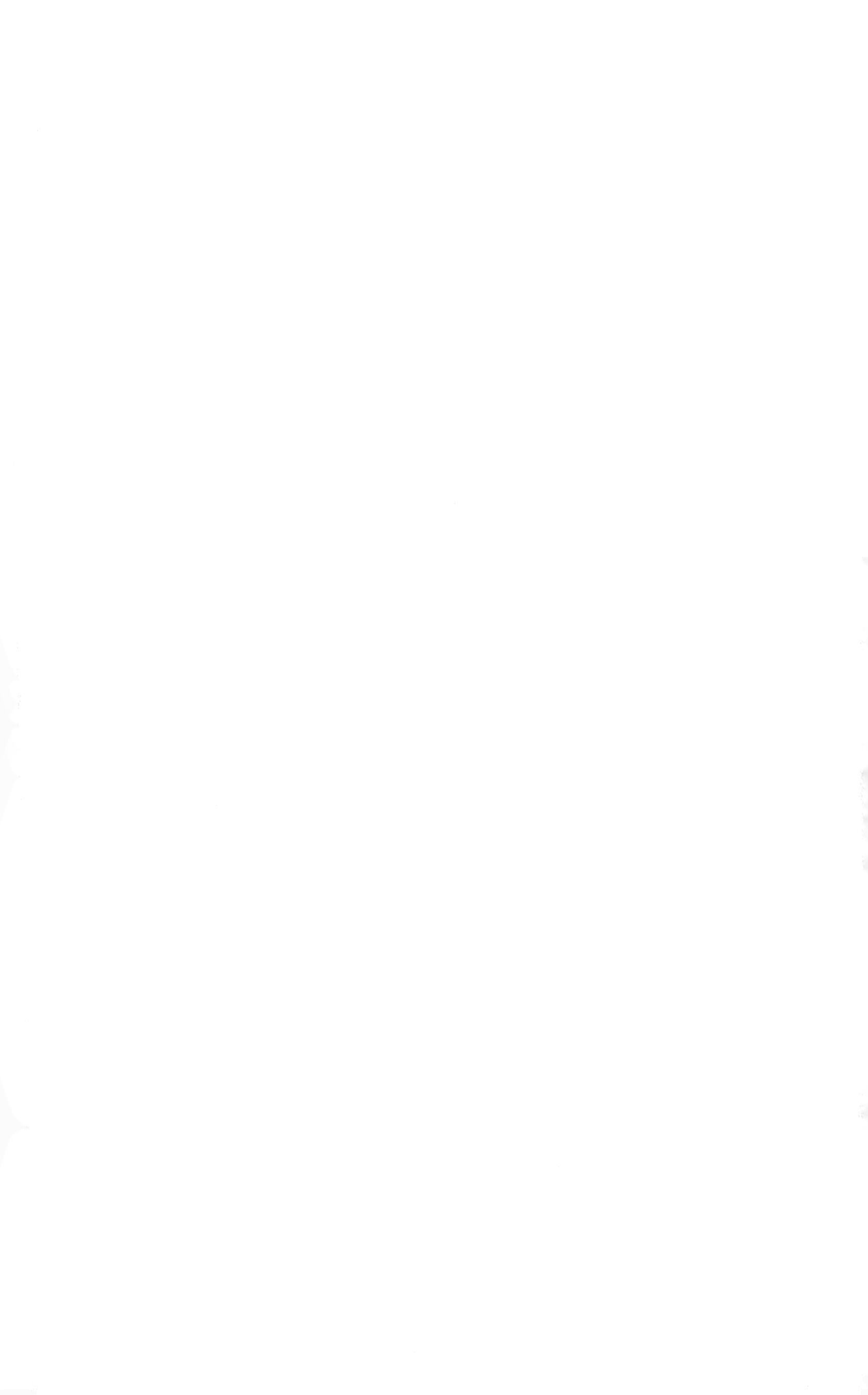

CPSIA information can be obtained
at www.ICGtesting.com
Printed in the USA
LVOW12s0728170716
496553LV00002B/2/P